Clinical Method

Clinical Method

A general practice approach

Third edition

Edited by

Robin C. Fraser, MD(Aberdeen), FRCGP

Professor of General Practice, University of Leicester;
General Practitioner, Leicester

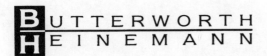

EDINBURGH LONDON NEW YORK OXFORD PHILADELPHIA ST LOUIS
SYDNEY TORONTO

Butterworth-Heinemann
An imprint of Elsevier Limited

First published 1987
Second edition 1992
    Reprinted 1993, 1994
Third edition 1999
    Reprinted 2000, 2001, 2002, 2003, 2005 (twice), 2006, 2007, 2008 (twice)

ISBN 978 0 7506 4005 3

British Library Cataloguing in Publication Data
A catalogue record for this book is available from the British Library

Library of Congress Cataloguing in Publication Data
A catalogue record for this book is available from the Library of Congress

your source for books,
journals and multimedia
in the health sciences
www.elsevierhealth.com

Working together to grow
libraries in developing countries
www.elsevier.com | www.bookaid.org | www.sabre.org

ELSEVIER   BOOK AID   Sabre Foundation
            International

The
publisher's
policy is to use
**paper manufactured
from sustainable forests**

Printed and bound in China

Contents

months presenting with a fever ● A retired gentleman with progressive shortness of breath ● A crying infant aged 5 weeks ● A child aged 7 years complaining of abdominal pain ● A man aged 27 years with low back pain ● A woman aged 38 years planning her marriage ● A man aged 40 years who has 'coughed up some blood' ● A woman aged 45 years who has been advised to have a hysterectomy ● Opportunities for anticipatory care in a man aged 29 years

11   **Assessing and enhancing consultation performance**   178
      Robin C. Fraser
      Introduction ● Essential components of educational assessment
      ● A systematic approach to assessing your own consultation
      performance: the practical steps ● Strategies to help overcome
      consultation weaknesses ● Key points ● References

      Appendix: The detailed contribution of general practice to   191
      undergraduate medical education and to the attributes
      of the independent practitioner

      Index   196

Preface to the first edition

Give me a fish and I eat for a day.
Teach me to fish and I eat for a lifetime.
Old Oriental saying

Even as long ago as 1925, it was realized that the undergraduate medical curriculum could not provide all the knowledge required to sustain a doctor throughout his or her professional lifetime (Flexner, 1925). Since that time, there has been a staggering increase in the volume of medical knowledge and it continues to grow at an accelerating rate. Nevertheless, there is still an overemphasis on the instillation and test of recall of factual knowledge in most medical schools (Pickering, 1978). According to one dean, medical students are: 'understretched but overwhelmed by the necessity to absorb a mass of facts' (Kessell, 1984), and within medical schools: 'learning too often takes precedence over reasoning' (Kaufman *et al.*, 1982).

It is, of course, essential for medical students to acquire a selective knowledge of facts, as is the mastery of certain motor skills (for example, the ability to conduct a competent physical examination or to use medical instruments). Nevertheless, greater emphasis must surely be placed on the development of cognitive skills (for example, the ability to think critically, to collect, transmit and evaluate information, and to act appropriately on it), along with the development of appropriate attitudes (for example, the recognition of the need to combine scientific and humanitarian values, and to respect the autonomy and personal dignity of the patient). In short, there is a need to instruct less and educate more in order to equip our future doctors with the ability to cope with the many changes which they will inevitably encounter during their professional careers.

This book has been written primarily for medical students. It has the immediate aim of helping them to gain maximum benefit from a period of exposure to, and teaching in, the setting of general practice as part of their basic medical education. More specifically it seeks to assist readers to recognize, adopt and develop those clinical skills and values that are fundamental to the practice of rational and humane clinical medicine, whatever the clinical setting. Although the authors have selected those aspects of clinical method that are best – but not necessarily exclusively – demonstrated in general practice (for further details *see* Appendix), the book is not narrowly vocational and it is intended to help all students to become better doctors, irrespective of their current career preference or eventual career choice.

The text concentrates on the principles of, and the concepts underlying, sound clinical method in its broadest sense, and provides guidance on how its many components need to be integrated and then applied in clinical practice for the benefit of patients. The authors have tried to avoid the use of jargon and, whenever possible, they have provided explanations and corroborative evidence for their stated views. Consequently, the book contains a fairly large number of annotated references.

By these means, it is hoped that readers will be helped towards a greater understanding of the fundamentals of clinical practice. As a consequence, they should become more aware of not only *how* to carry out a particular clinical activity, but also – and most importantly – *why* it should be carried out at all or in a particular way. This, in turn, should lead to an increased capability to identify, manage and sometimes solve new and unfamiliar problems through a process of systematic and critical appraisal, instead of relying on guesswork or memory alone.

Although primarily directed at medical students, the book is also likely to prove useful to trainee general practitioners because it should help them to bridge the considerable gap between the differing styles and content of clinical medicine as practised in the respective settings of hospital and primary care.

It should be noted that, throughout this book, the masculine gender will be used for the sake of convenience.

Robin C. Fraser
Leicester, 1987

References

Flexner, A. (1925). *Medical Education*. London: Macmillan.

Kaufman, A., Kleeper, D., Obenshain, S. S. *et al.* (1982). Undergraduate medical education for primary care: a case study in New Mexico. *Southern Medical Journal*, 75, 1110.

Kessell, N. (1984). Conference of Medical Academic Representatives (editorial report). *British Medical Journal*, 288, 1929.

Pickering, G. (1978). *The Quest for Excellence in Medical Education*. Oxford: Oxford University Press.

Preface to the second edition

Although every effort has been made to preserve the essential content and character of the first edition, a number of changes have been made. Three completely new chapters have been introduced (Chapter 2, The consultation; Chapter 8, Clinical problem-solving and patient management; some practical scenarios, and Chapter 9, Ethics in practice). The opportunity has also been taken to update and revise certain sections of all the other chapters in the light of developments since the first edition. The chapter on 'The doctor as counsellor' has been removed, although some collated extracts are included in Chapter 4.

The book is again primarily directed at medical students. Nevertheless, my fellow authors and I were pleased that the first edition had a good reception not only from medical students but also from vocational trainees, both in the UK and beyond. We hope that the second edition will prove to be even more useful.

All the authors would like to acknowledge the assistance given by the following in the preparation of the book: the many authors and publishers who readily gave permission for their work to be reproduced or quoted; past and present colleagues and students in the Department of General Practice, University of Leicester, for helpful comments and suggestions; Mrs Patricia Manno, Departmental Secretary, who attended to all the secretarial duties so willingly and efficiently; the Department of Audio-Visual Services, University of Leicester, for drawing Figures 1.1, 1.2, 1.4, 3.3, 3.4 and 6.1; and Sue Deeley, Senior Commissioning Editor, and the staff of Butterworth-Heinemann for their professional support.

Robin C. Fraser
Leicester, 1992

Preface to the third edition

Since the publication of the second edition of this book in 1992, three major developments have occurred to affect clinical practice and education. These are the growing acceptance and influence of evidence-based medicine, the increased role of the doctor in advising patients to make health-related lifestyle changes, and new recommendations on undergraduate medical education (General Medical Council, 1993). The GMC decreed that the acquisition of basic clinical methods should be a priority, that students should take more responsibility for their own learning and that more teaching should be moved out of hospitals into the community. Although previous editions of this book did address all these issues, the third edition has been structured and extended to reflect them even more.

Two completely new chapters have been introduced (Chapter 8, A systematic approach in the consultation to lifestyle modification: helping patients to stop smoking, and Chapter 11, Assessing and enhancing consultation performance). In addition, a third chapter (Chapter 10) has been totally reconstructed and extended to provide 11 new clinical challenges, containing a total of 34 questions, compared to eight challenges and 18 questions in the second edition. This is aimed to provide the reader with more opportunities for self-assessment.

Nevertheless, the temptation to make changes just for the sake of change has been resisted. Although all the other eight chapters have been revised and updated as appropriate, the underlying principles and concepts are unchanged – and unchanging. Accordingly, my fellow authors and I hope that the book will continue to be positively received by medical students and by doctors in training, both in the UK and beyond – although the book is still primarily directed at medical students.

Again, my fellow authors and I would like to acknowledge the contributions made by the following in the preparation of this book: the many authors and publishers who readily gave permission for their work to be reproduced or quoted; past and present colleagues and students in the Department of General Practice and Primary Health Care, University of Leicester, for helpful comments and suggestions; Mrs Patricia Manno, Departmental Secretary, who once again attended to all the secretarial duties so enthusiastically and efficiently; and the staff of Butterworth-Heinemann for their professional support.

Robin C. Fraser
Leicester, 1998

Reference

General Medical Council (1993). Tomorrow's Doctors. *Recommendations on Undergraduate Medical Education*. London: General Medical Council.

Contributors

Gary E. Aram, MB, ChB(Liverpool), MRCGP, DCH, DObst RCOG
Lecturer in General Practice, University of Leicester; General Practitioner, Countesthorpe, Leicestershire

Timothy J. Coleman, MD(Leicester), MRCGP
Lecturer in General Practice, University of Leicester; General Practitioner, Leicester

Robin C. Fraser, MD(Aberdeen), FRCGP
Professor of General Practice, University of Leicester; General Practitioner, Leicester

Brian R. McAvoy, BSc, MB, ChB(Glasgow), MD(Leicester), FRCP, FRCGP, MRNZCGP
William Leech Professor of Primary Health Care, University of Newcastle-upon-Tyne; formerly Elaine Gurr Professor of General Practice, University of Auckland, New Zealand and Senior Lecturer in General Practice, University of Leicester

Pauline A. McAvoy, MB, ChB(Glasgow), MRNZCGP
Chief Executive, Gateshead and South Tyneside Health Authority. Formerly Senior Lecturer in General Practice, University of Auckland, New Zealand and Lecturer in General Practice, University of Leicester

Robert K. McKinley, BSc, MD(Belfast), MRCP, FRCGP
Senior Lecturer in General Practice, University of Leicester; General Practitioner, Leicester

M. Elan Preston-Whyte, MB, BCh(Wales), FRCGP, DA
Lecturer in General Practice, University of Leicester

1
Setting the scene

Robin C. Fraser

Primary care is the point of entry into the health
services system and the locus of responsibility for
organizing care for patients and populations over
time. There is a universally held belief that the
substance of primary care is essentially simple.
Nothing could be further from the truth
(Starfield, 1992).

This chapter will describe the role of the general practitioner, outline the
flavour and content of general practice, and highlight some of the ways in
which these differ from clinical practice in the hospital setting. It will also
provide some background information to enable you to become more
familiar with the health status of the community and patterns of patient
illness behaviour, since general practice is that level of care between self-
and hospital-care.

The information presented in this chapter has been selected to help
to make the reader rapidly more aware of the very different nature and
range of diagnostic probabilities in general as compared to hospital
practice. This is a prerequisite for the development of a doctor's ability
to recognize and manage clinical problems in the setting of general
practice, since so much clinical judgement – whether in hospital or
general practice – starts from an awareness of the context of the clinical
task and its associated probabilities. You will already be aware of the
extent to which clinical perspectives need to be adjusted even when
moving from a paediatric to an adult medical setting in hospital. Still
greater adjustments to the basic clinical approach are required in dealing
with patients in the orthopaedic or gynaecological departments. The
'culture shock' in moving from hospital to general practice, however, is
likely to be the greatest you will experience.

In clinical practice in any setting, moreover, the ability to generate
appropriate diagnostic hypotheses rests not only on knowledge of crude
probabilities: the learner must also be aware of how these crude
probabilities are influenced in a complex way by a variety of other
factors, such as the nature and duration of presenting symptoms and the
particular characteristics of patients affected by them (see Chapter 3).
Nowhere is this truer than in primary care.

Furthermore, in this setting it is especially important to have some understanding of the context in which medical and other problems with an impact on health arise – and how people react to them – in order to develop the necessary skills not only to identify them, but also to manage them appropriately. Indeed it has been demonstrated that a general practitioner's knowledge of patients' social problems influences management decisions in 17% of all consultations, with stressful working conditions being the most frequent influence (Gulbrandsen *et al.*, 1998). When the main reason for the consultation is 'psychological' or 'social', this proportion increases to 67% and 55%, respectively (see Chapter 4).

No attempt should be made to memorize the individual percentages listed in this chapter; they are provided to give the reader a 'feel' for the frequency of occurrence of a whole range of phenomena in terms of orders of magnitude rather than detail. It should also be borne in mind that very large variations can occur in the attributes and activities of particular general practices. The practice to which you are attached, therefore, may differ quite substantially from the average figures quoted in the second part of this chapter depending on its particular characteristics – for example, its geographical location, the social class structure of the population it serves and, not least, the attitudes and clinical behaviours of the doctors themselves.

Community morbidity and patient illness behaviour

The general practitioner is normally the patient's first point of contact with organized medical services; furthermore, the consultation is made at the patient's instigation. Consequently, general practitioners must be aware not only of patterns of illness in the community (Table 1.1) but must also understand the variety of ways in which people react when they perceive themselves to be ill (Table 1.2). The range of reactions is referred to as 'patient illness behaviour', which has been defined by Mechanic (1961) as:

> The way in which given symptoms may be differently perceived, evaluated and acted upon – or not acted upon – by different kinds of people.

Table 1.1   State of health of the general population

State of health	Population (%)
Healthy	13
Not ill	52
Ill	18
Chronic sickness	12
Disabled	5

From Kohn and White, 1976.

Table 1.2   Reactions to symptoms and problems

Reaction	Numbers (%)
Taking no action	43
Self-medication (over the counter)	36
Consult general practitioner	13
Home remedy	8

Adapted from Fry, 1993.

It is readily apparent from these tables that only a small proportion of the population is free of symptoms or feels healthy at any point in time. At the other end of the spectrum, however, only a small minority of the population suffers from chronic sickness or disablement. The bulk of the population at any point in time will experience symptoms which are sufficient to disturb their overall sense of being healthy without making them feel ill, but which do not inevitably result in a consultation with a doctor. Thus, a significant 'clinical iceberg' exists, to which self-care is the dominant response (Figure 1.1). The consequence is that, on any single day, 33% of the population are self-medicating and 33% are taking prescribed medication (Fry, 1993). Table 1.3 lists the commonest symptoms resulting in self-medication. It has been demonstrated, however, that consultation rates among people

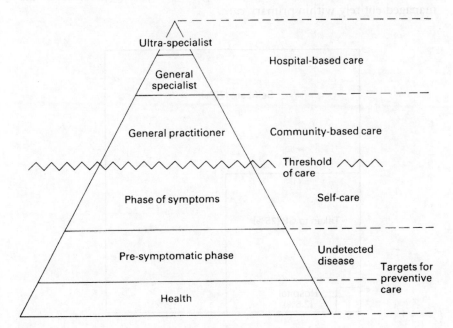

Figure 1.1   The clinical iceberg and levels of care

Table 1.3 Commonest symptoms resulting in self-medication

Symptom	Self-medication (%)*
Tiredness	35
Headache	30
Aches and pains	25
Overweight	20
Backache	15
Others	30

* Often there is more than one reason for self-medication.
From Fry, 1993.

who self-initiate drug treatment are lower, thus implying that self-medication is used as an alternative, rather than an addition, to seeking professional medical advice (Dunnel and Cartwright, 1972). On the other hand, self-medication that fails to remove the symptoms is often followed by a consultation with a general practitioner.

Figure 1.2 represents a collation of the findings of a number of studies, which indicates that only one person in every four who experiences symptoms decides to cross the threshold between self-care and professional care by consulting a general practitioner. Of those, only one in ten is subsequently referred to hospital. It should be noted, therefore, that most episodes of illness presenting to the general practitioner are managed entirely within primary care.

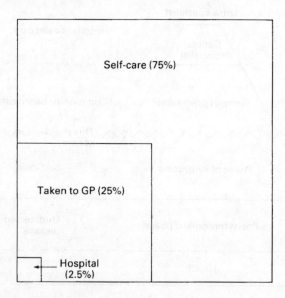

Figure 1.2 Levels of care of symptoms

Factors that influence the decision to consult

The factors that influence an individual's decision to seek professional medical advice are many and varied. Indeed, Becker (1979) has described the influencing factors as:

a constellation of diverse and complex health-related attitudes and behaviours which often appear to be enigmatic, irrational, erroneous and relatively immutable.

Furthermore, because identical factors have a differential impact on individuals, there is also a wide variation in help-seeking behaviour. One consequence is that some people who would benefit from seeking professional help do not do so, and vice versa. What is clear, however, is that the decision to seek medical care does *not* closely correlate with the possible seriousness of the symptoms experienced by the potential patient. As Robinson (1971) has pointed out:

Neither the presence nor the obviousness of the symptom, neither the medical seriousness nor the objective disability, seem to differentiate those symptoms which do and those which do not get [i.e. are not brought for] professional treatment.

Many patients, for example, do not appreciate the importance of certain symptoms that could indicate underlying malignant disease. It has been shown that only 50% of women were aware that post-menopausal bleeding could be a symptom of cancer, and only 57% of women realized that a painless breast lump could be malignant (Walker, 1982).

Zola (1973) and others have established that the basic reason for many consultations is not that a patient has a disease. Moreover, Zola concluded that the factors influencing health action are mainly social and psychological in nature, rather than physiological, anatomical or bio-chemical. There are, however, some identifiable influences on the decision taken by people whether or not to consult. These include, for example, the nature or perceived threat of the symptom or symptom complex, whether the symptoms involve an adult or child, and the potential patient's social class or ethnicity.

Table 1.4 indicates the differential extent to which individuals are prepared to tolerate a range of symptoms without consulting a general practitioner. Vague and familiar symptoms such as tiredness and headache are best tolerated and most likely to be dealt with through self-medication (see also Table 1.3). It is likely that pain in the chest is least well tolerated because of its potentially serious implications, whereas a disinclination to tolerate a sore throat is more likely to be related to the immediacy of the unpleasant impact of the symptom itself.

Table 1.4   Likelihood of symptoms leading to consultation

Symptoms	Ratio of symptom episodes to consultation
Changes in energy	456:1
Headache	184:1
Disturbance of gastric function	109:1
Backache	52:1
Pain in lower limb	49:1
Emotional/psychological	46:1
Abdominal pain	29:1
Disturbance of menstruation	20:1
Sore throat	18:1
Pain in chest	14:1

From Banks *et al.*, 1975.

Lydeard and Jones (1989) have provided definitive evidence that the perceived threat of an otherwise tolerable symptom can be the principal reason for a consultation. In their study on patients with dyspepsia, they reported statistically significant differences in the belief among consulters compared to non-consulters that their symptoms could lead to a serious or fatal condition (74% v. 17% respectively); stomach cancer (29% v. 13%), cancer generally (55% v. 30%) or heart disease (66% v. 35%). Thus, concern about the potentially serious implications of their symptoms took precedence over the severity or frequency of symptoms or the presence of associated symptoms in influencing the patient's decision to consult. It should also be remembered, however, that in some instances the perceived threat of a particular symptom or sign may mitigate against seeking medical help because of a fear that a person's underlying suspicions might be confirmed by the doctor.

Wilkin *et al.* (1987a) pointed out that the threshold for consultation is lower in children than in adults. In assessing the likelihood of adults consulting a general practitioner with a range of symptoms, they established that only 17% would be likely or very likely to consult with 'a heavy cold with a slight temperature'. On the other hand, the figures in parentheses indicate the extent to which it would be likely or very likely that the same adults would bring their children to a doctor with similar symptoms: earache (79%), temperature (60%) and sore throat (55%).

Table 1.5 shows the differential impact of another set of symptoms and signs on the perceived need for medical attention, and how this is influenced in turn by social class. It is evident that, for all symptoms and signs, there is a gradient in the perceived need to seek medical attention from the upper to the lower social classes, the former being much more likely to seek medical attention for any given symptom or sign.

Table 1.5   Social class, symptoms and perceived need for medical attention

Symptom/sign	Social class (%)*		
	Upper	Middle	Lower
Blood in urine	100	93	69
Blood in stool	98	89	60
Lump in breast	94	71	44
Excessive vaginal bleeding	92	83	54
Lump in abdomen	92	65	34
Fainting spells	80	51	33
Loss of weight	80	51	21
Pain in chest	80	51	31
Persistent headaches	80	56	22
Continued coughing	77	78	23
Shortness of breath	77	55	21
Swelling of ankles	77	76	23
Persistent backache	53	44	19

* Figures given are the percentages of symptom episodes that lead to consultations.
From Koos, 1954. Copyright © 1954 Columbia University Press, by permission.

Another social variable that exerts a strong influence on whether or not to consult is ethnicity. In one study it was noted that 56% of Asian adults with headache consulted their general practitioners compared to 24% of non-Asians; with regard to the symptom of tiredness, the respective figures were 33% and 12% (Rashid and Jagger, 1996). In addition to those factors considered above, there are a number of other factors which are more likely to lead an individual to make the decision to consult a doctor. These are, in no particular sequence of importance:

1. An acute rather than a gradual onset of symptoms
2. Symptoms which interfere with social activity
3. Symptoms with greater frequency and persistence, given a similar level of severity
4. Bizarre symptoms
5. Visible signs
6. Pressure from relatives, friends or work colleagues
7. Being elderly, female, divorced/separated or lonely
8. Previous experience of similar symptoms that require health care
9. A good doctor – patient relationship
10. An unrelated personal crisis.

Clinical applications

The patients encountered in general practice, therefore, are there on the basis of lay, highly individualistic judgements, whereas the patients encountered in hospital practice have principally arrived there following a professional decision-making process, usually undertaken by a general practitioner. As a consequence, the symptoms patients present to general practitioners tend to be 'unorganized' whereas those presented in hospital tend to be more 'medicalized'.

Because the patient decides *when* to consult, it is also particularly important for the primary care doctor – as an integral and early part of the process of clinical problem-solving – to discover *why* the patient has so decided. If the general practitioner can detect the true reason for the patient consulting, the diagnosis is likely to be more accurate and subsequent management will likewise be more appropriate.

Furthermore, the doctor needs to bear in mind the enormous disparity in levels of awareness that exists in the general population concerning health matters. On the one hand, it has been shown that many patients are unaware of the correct location of the major body organs (Rashid and Jagger, 1996). For example, 25% do not know where the heart is located, and figures for other organs are as follows: stomach 50%, liver 75%, lungs 40%. Five per cent of the population are not even aware of where the brain can be found in the body! At the other end of the scale, many patients 'hold elaborate and often sophisticated theories of their own illness' (Armstrong, 1991). Accordingly the general practitioner, as doctor of first contact, has a special requirement to tailor an approach to suit the particular needs and levels of awareness of each individual patient.

Unfortunately for doctors, the decision to seek medical care does *not* occur at a uniformly recognized and predictable threshold, nor does it correlate closely with the potential seriousness of the symptoms experienced by the patient. A symptom that would be recognized by a doctor as potentially serious may remain unrecognized or be totally ignored by some patients. Doctors cannot assume, for example, that women who present with post-menopausal bleeding, or even a breast lump, will all share the doctor's awareness that these presentations could be caused by cancer. With such patients, therefore, a particularly sensitive approach is required.

On the other hand, some patients consult with relatively trivial symptoms as a consequence of holding erroneous views as to what constitutes good health. For example, two-thirds of people in the UK believe that a daily bowel movement is necessary to be healthy. As a consequence, it is likely that any deviation from this pattern will result in either self-medication or a consultation, which may be seen as unnecessary by the doctor but very necessary by the patient. This is a potential recipe for conflict, unless the doctor establishes that the reason for the consultation is a mistaken belief on the part of the patient that constipation is the problem. Consequently, a mixture of reassurance and health education becomes the appropriate response, rather than dietary advice, the prescribing of a laxative, an unnecessary rectal examination or a display of irritation. By the same token, many parents bring their children principally for reassurance and an explanation of their symptoms, rather than for medication; doctors should respond accordingly.

Patients may also consult because they have reached the limit of tolerating a particular symptom, or because they are worried by the possible significance of a symptom. It is essential that the doctor determines which of these is the particular stimulus for the consultation, for the following reasons. There is little point in providing a patient who presents with back pain with an analgesic if the sole reason for the consultation is a wish for reassurance that the backache is not a symptom of cancer; conversely, there is no point in reassuring a patient with backache that it is not cancer if the thought had never entered the patient's head, and what is wanted is pain relief to make work possible. Furthermore, there is little to be gained by suggesting paracetamol for pain relief if the patient has already self-medicated with the same drug and found it ineffective; in this case, the credibility – and, therefore, the effectiveness – of the doctor will be damaged because of the failure to establish whether self-medication had already occurred. Self-medication is so common, the doctor should always enquire about it. Also, because patterns of illness behaviour vary greatly from one individual to another, doctors need to be aware that:

> one disease may be manifest among a group of patients in widely divergent ways, and that illness as experienced by patients may be as highly individualized as fingerprints (Tarlov, 1988).

Nevertheless, general practitioners can often recognize specific triggers to seeking medical advice in particular patients because of their continuing contact with their patients over long periods of time – for example, those who consult with vague physical symptoms on the anniversary of the death of a loved one when all they want is a chat and to be cheered up. Furthermore, many patients produce a recognizable and repeating pattern of physical symptoms as a reaction to stress, often amounting to a personal hallmark. Although it is important not to label patients too rigidly, an awareness of recurring patterns of illness behaviour in individuals can enable doctors to make a more appropriate – and usually more effective – response.

It should also be remembered that some patients choose to present to their doctor with a minor – and usually physical – symptom as a 'ticket of admission', when their real wish is to raise a deeper and/or more serious problem. A variant of this approach is when patients state, often as they are about to leave the consulting room, 'While I'm here, doctor, I'd like to mention . . .'. By these approaches, patients can 'test out' their doctor before venturing to divulge the real reason for the consultation. This is often referred to as a patient's 'hidden agenda', and this will not usually be forthcoming if the doctor fails to meet the patient's initial expectations.

Finally, owing to all the reasons stated above, it should always be borne in mind that:

> The physician should understand why and when a person seeks medical attention, how he views his own sickness, how he reports his symptoms and interprets his feelings, and what changes in his life occur because of his illness or treatment. The factors are always influenced by the respective cultural backgrounds of patient and physician (Jaco, 1958).

The nature and content of general practice

There are approximately 33 000 NHS general practitioners in the United Kingdom, most of whom work in groups of three or four doctors, with less than 10% in 'single-handed' practice. Of the total population, 98% are registered with an individual general practitioner of their choice, and each NHS practitioner has an average of approximately 1850 registered patients. Almost 80% of these consult their doctor one or more times each year and over 90% consult within a period of 5 years. The average annual consultation rate per patient is between three and four times per year, although it is higher in females (4.4) than males (3.3) and also at the extremes of age (Figure 1.3). The average NHS general practitioner will conduct some 30–40 surgery consultations and make three or four home visits daily; these activities will occupy some 68% of the working day. The rest of the time is taken up with the provision of additional patient services such as correspondence, telephone calls, preparing repeat prescriptions, consulting with partners and specialists, administration and clinical audit (Fry, 1993). Increasingly, general practitioners are also undertaking activities such as child surveillance and minor surgery as part of their day-to-day work.

Most general practitioners work in close association with a range of other health and allied professionals such as nurses, health visitors, midwives and social workers – often collectively referred to as members of the primary health care team. Additional members of the team such as dieticians, counsellors and chiropodists can be found in a minority of practices. Increasingly, team members are housed under the same roof, often in purpose-built premises. More practices are also employing their own nurses to assist in health promotion clinics and routine annual assessment of patients aged over 75 years.

Nevertheless, the nature of general practice is changing all the time. For example, it has been speculated that, into 'the new millenium', even greater evolution of general practice will occur:

> All the district's GPs and their teams [will] practise from well-equipped family health centres, which co-operate with one another to provide 24-hour emergency cover with several strategically placed out-of-hours walk-in centres, complete with community pharmacies. These are

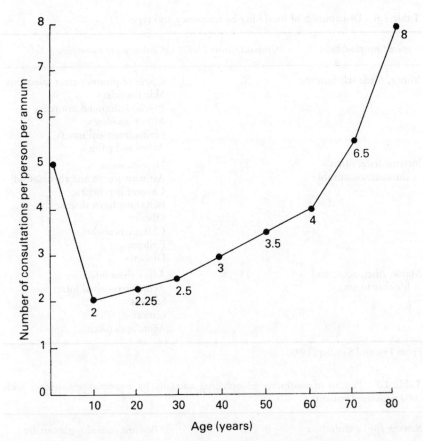

Figure 1.3   Doctor attendance rates and patient age (from Fry, 1993)

supplemented by GP and nurse-led telephone information and advice services for patients who are unsure whether they should go to the Accident and Emergency Department or whether they can safely treat themselves until they can see their own doctor (Rigge, 1998).

Tables 1.6 to 1.8 indicate the wide range of clinical events and social pathology encountered in general practice. It is evident from these tables that the general practitioner deals mainly with common diseases and problems, many of which are transient and self-limiting and some of which are chronic. Major diseases are uncommon, with only eight new cancers a year per general practitioner, six acute abdomens, six strokes and six myocardial infarctions.

Thus, the nature and spectrum of diseases encountered in general practice – and to which you will be exposed during practice attachment – contrasts sharply with the hospital patterns of morbidity with which you will be more familiar (Figure 1.4). For example:

Table 1.6 Distribution of morbidity by frequency and type

Type of morbidity	Consultations (%)	Commonest examples
Minor, often self-limiting	52	Upper respiratory tract infections Skin disorders Psycho-emotional disorders Minor accidents Gastrointestinal upsets Aches and pains
Intermediate, often chronic/non-curable	33	Hypertension Arthritis (osteo and rheumatoid) Chronic psychiatric Ischaemic heart disease Obesity Chronic bronchitis Epilepsy Diabetes
Major, often acute and life-threatening	15	Acute chest infection Acute myocardial infarction Strokes Cancer Acute appendicitis

From Fry and Sandler, 1993.

Table 1.7 Pattern of morbidity encountered annually by a general practitioner with 2000 registered patients

Reason for consultation	Persons consulting annually
Preventive procedures (immunisations, screening, 'check-ups', family planning, travel advice, etc.)	800
Acute upper respiratory infections	500
Neuroses	130
Skin diseases	125
Arthritis	120
Back problems	120
Rheumatism	100
Hypertension	85
Asthma	85
Hay fever	56
'Pneumonia and flu'	47
Angina	23
Migraine	23
Diabetes	22
Heart failure	18
Malignant neoplasms	15
Thyroid disorders	13
Acute myocardial infarction	6
Acute appendicitis	2

From Fry, 1993.

Table 1.8   Social pathology

Condition	Likely number per 2000 patients
Poverty (grants)	300
Unemployed	90
One parent families	30
Marriages	13
Homeless ('official')	5
Divorces	5
Terminations of pregnancy	5
Crime	
Burglaries	35
Drunken drivers	5
In prison	2
Sexual assault	1

From Fry and Sandler, 1993.

1. Whereas domestic problems and simple anxiety states are managed almost entirely within general practice, it is interesting to note that the presence of somatic symptoms makes hospital referral of neurosis more likely. This probably reflects a concern – often shared by both patient and doctor – that underlying physical disease be excluded.
2. Although respiratory disorders are very prevalent in general practice, these consist mostly of acute, often self-limiting conditions. The acute stages of the more serious, but less common, respiratory conditions are managed mainly in the hospital setting, having been initially recognized in general practice, where aftercare will also be provided.
3. The greatest contrast occurs in respect of malignant diseases, which are relatively rare in general practice (Table 1.9) but are commonly encountered in hospital, as virtually all patients with cancer are referred.

Nevertheless, the impact of particular conditions in general practice, in terms of the clinical effort that needs to be mounted to cope with them, is often inversely proportional to their frequency of occurrence. For example, a patient with a malignant disease will require an average of 12 doctor contacts per episode of disease per annum, whereas a patient who has an upper respiratory tract infection will require less than two consultations per episode (Davis, 1975). It may appear, therefore, that malignant disease is commoner in general practice than is actually the case.

The list of symptoms with which patients most commonly present in general practice (Table 1.10) reveals the rich variety of diagnostic problems encountered, although musculoskeletal, respiratory, skin, and

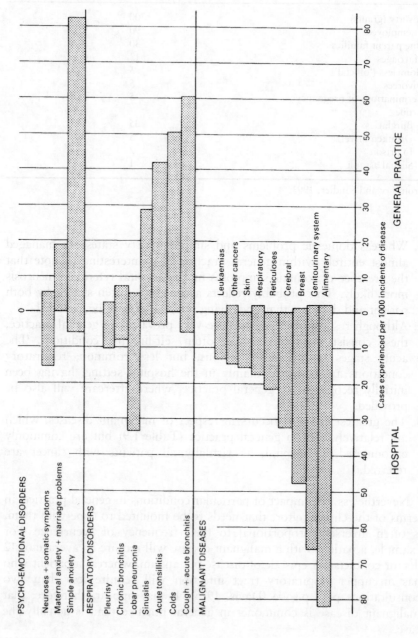

Figure 1.4 Experience of disease: hospital versus general practice (from Hodgkin, 1978)

Table 1.9   Selected cancer inception rates per 2000 general practice patients

New cancer site	Inception rate
All cancers	8 in 1 year
Lung, skin, breast	1 each in 1 year
Stomach, rectum, prostate, bladder	1 each in 3 years
Colon	2 in 3 years
Pancreas, ovary, lymphoma	1 each in 5 years
Leukaemia	1 in 6 years
Cervix	1 in 7 years
Uterus	1 in 9 years
Oesophagus, melanoma	1 each in 10 years
Myeloma	1 in 12 years
Testes	1 in 15 years
Thyroid	1 in 25 years

From Fry and Sandler, 1993.

Table 1.10   Commonest presenting symptoms

Symptom	Frequency (%)
Muscular aches	13.2
Cough	11.1
Skin infection/irritation	7.9
Abdominal pain	5.5
Diarrhoea/vomiting	4.7
Sore throat/inflamed tonsils	4.6
Cold/blocked nose/sinus	4.5
Back pain	3.9
Breathlessness/wheezing	3.1
Chest pain	2.9

Adapted from Wilkin et al. (1987b).

gastrointestinal symptoms are the most prominent. Wilkin et al. (1987b) found that 23 presenting symptoms accounted for 87% of consultations. In addition to those listed in Table 1.10, the others were: headache (2.6%), dizziness (2.5%), tired/unwell (2.4%), ear infection/ pain (2.3%), depression (2%), anxiety/nervousness (2%), urinary tract problems (1.9%), menstrual problems (1.9%), vaginal problems (1.9%), eye infection/irritation (1.7%), fever/chill (1.6%), hearing problem (1.2%), and sleep disturbance (1.0%).

The relative frequencies with which particular diagnoses result from the presenting symptom of cough are detailed in Table 1.11. It is evident that the most likely underlying causes relate to the upper respiratory tract, and only rarely will a life-threatening cause be responsible. This contrasts sharply with the likely diagnostic outcomes in referred patients

Table 1.11   Diagnostic probability: presenting symptom of cough ($N = 527$)

Diagnosis made	Frequency (%)	Crude probability
Acute bronchitis	36	Most likely
Common cold	35	
Influenza	7	Less likely
Chronic bronchitis	6	
Laryngitis tracheitis	6	
Pneumonia	1.9	
Whooping cough	0.7	
Measles	0.4	
Pulmonary tuberculosis	0.4	Rare
Carcinoma of lung	0.2	
Other	7	

Adapted from Morrell, 1976, reproduced by kind permission of the author.

with cough presenting in a hospital chest clinic, when a much higher proportion of serious underlying disease would be expected.

Figure 1.5 provides a detailed contrast between the underlying causes of chest pain in patients presenting in hospital and general practice, respectively. This again highlights the differing range of probabilities and the associated levels of severity between the two settings.

It should also be remembered that patients with psychiatric and emotional disorders might also initially present with physical symptoms. This occurs because some patients fail to recognize the true underlying cause of their symptoms, and some patients do recognize the likely underlying cause as emotional but feel that the presentation of physical

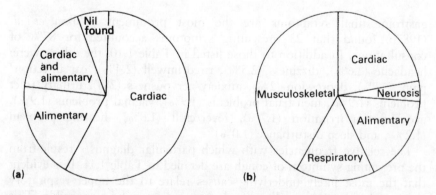

Figure 1.5   Contrasting causes of chest pain presenting in: (a) hospital (from Bennett and Atkinson, 1966) and (b) general practice (from Frank, 1970)

symptoms is more acceptable to doctors. Indeed, Morrell (1976) calculated that emotional disorders comprised the single commonest explanation for the presenting symptom of headache, accounting for almost 20% of all causes. Furthermore, many presentations consist of multiple symptoms and problems, which can make the task of problem identification and diagnosis infinitely more difficult. It has been estimated that the average number of problems presented in a general practice consultation is 2.5 (Bentsen, 1976).

It is evident, therefore, that the range, type, severity and frequency of problems encountered in general practice are very different from those in hospital. Consequently, you will be required to reorient your clinical thoughts – and your clinical approach – to this new context. The data presented above indicate that most symptoms and problems encountered in general practice do not result in 'serious' diseases in the conventional sense, since they pose little threat to life. Nevertheless, they can be responsible for much disability and great unhappiness. They also support the adage that 'common diseases occur most commonly', although it is important to remember that rare diseases *do* occur in general practice and need to be considered, when appropriate, in generating diagnostic hypotheses (see Chapter 3).

The contrasting roles of the general practitioner and hospital specialist

In keeping with the substantial differences in the structure and content of general and hospital practice, differences also exist between the professional roles and attitudes of general practitioners and hospital specialists.

In drawing attention to these differences (summarized in Table 1.12), it is important to make clear that no attempt is being made to suggest that one form of care is superior or inferior to the other. Both are to be equally valued, and both are essential. Nor is it being suggested that general practitioners have a monopoly of caring attitudes and hospital specialists a monopoly of scientific rigour. Whatever the setting, a good bedside manner is no substitute for clinical competence, as Barber (1956) pointed out:

> I would rather be in the hands of a man with an accurate knowledge of medicine and with but little of the milk of human kindness, than in the hands of the kindest man imaginable who did not really know his job.

As a corollary, 'clever' doctors will be handicapped in bringing their skills to bear if they are unable to make their patients trust or believe in them. Consequently, all clinicians, whether in hospital or general

Table 1.12   Differences between general practice and hospital

General practice – practitioner	Hospital – specialist
Structure	
Cares for a small registered population (2000)	Cares for a large unregistered population (250 000+)
Patients registered with individual doctor	No registration system
Patients have direct access	Access usually via GP
Situated close to patient's home	Situated far from most patients' homes
Huge variability between practices (e.g. age, social class of patients, geographical distribution)	Hospitals exhibit far less variability
Function	
Responsibility for all *health* care for patient	Responsibility for specialty-related *medical* care
Responsibility for all presenting problems irrespective of age, sex or morbidity	Responsibility for specialty-related problems only: restricted by age (e.g. paediatrics) or sex (obs. & gynae.)
Presented with undifferentiated problems/diseases	Presented with more organized disease
Deals with common diseases and social problems	Deals mainly with rare diseases or atypical versions of common diseases
Makes infrequent and highly selective use of 'high technology'	Makes frequent and less selective use of 'high technology'
Continuing responsibility for patients	Episodic responsibility for patients
Repeated opportunities for anticipatory care	Fewer opportunities for anticipatory care
Attitudes	
'Whole person' oriented: uses 'triple diagnosis'	Disease oriented: usually either physical *or* psychological
Prepared to use time as diagnostic tool (nice to know)	Little use of time as diagnostic tool (need to know)
Importance of doctor–patient relationship and its uses recognized and valued	Doctor–patient relationship less well demonstrated or used
If no cure, recognizes need for continuing care and support	If no cure, the patient is often discharged
Patient's viewpoint and autonomy recognized	Less recognition of patient's viewpoint and autonomy

practice, need to master the scientific and humanitarian aspects of the practice of medicine, although there are clinical circumstances in which one or the other may, quite legitimately, predominate.

> In the moment to moment challenges of the intensive care unit, technical skills and emergency decision making are more important than communication skills. In the ambulatory setting, personal factors of empathy, communication and patient education are far more needed – and much less taught (Federman, 1990).

The task of the general practitioner is to provide personal, primary, preventive and continuing care to individuals, families and a practice population. The care provided is also comprehensive, since it is given irrespective of patients' age or sex, or the type of illnesses they have or believe they have. In contrast, the hospital specialist has responsibility for specialty-related problems only, and may be further restricted by the age of the patient (as in paediatrics and geriatrics) or by the sex of the patient (as in gynaecology). Although dealing with a narrower spectrum of disease, however, the hospital specialist has a greater depth of knowledge and skill relating to that particular specialty than the general practitioner.

Moreover, general practitioners' responsibilities are limited to a much smaller and relatively static population for which they will provide continuing care – often in the patients' own homes – over many years. It is known, for example, that over 40% of a general practitioner's patients remain registered with that general practitioner for 20 years or more (Ritchie *et al.*, 1981). Many general practitioners will be providing care simultaneously for several generations of the same family; indeed, many will be providing care for children whose parents they had delivered a generation previously. Such a shared heritage greatly facilitates the consultation process for both doctor and patient, and it is well recognized that consultations in general practice are less formal and more intimate than they tend to be in hospital. The hospital doctor, on the other hand, is limited to episodic responsibility for patients and is rarely, if ever, in a position to provide care for a whole family.

Perhaps the most distinctive attribute of the general practitioner, according to McWhinney (1975), is that:

> His commitment is to people more than to a body of knowledge or a branch of technology.

McWhinney was at pains to point out that the term 'commitment to people' went beyond having an interest in, or a concern for, people – attributes which all clinicians, whether in hospital or general practice, should possess. As McWhinney observed, however, the doctor who has a commitment to people finds that:

> Problems become interesting and important not only for their own sake but because they are Mr. Smith's or Mrs. Jones' problems. Very often in such relations there is not even a very clear distinction between a medical problem and a non-medical one.

Nevertheless, it is essential that doctors should not become so keen to see their patients as people that they forget to treat them as patients – to their potential detriment (MacNaughton, 1998).

Because of a combination of the factors listed above, general practitioners are more likely to form much closer personal relationships with
their patients than is normally possible for a hospital doctor. A feature
of general practice is the frequency with which such relationships are
used professionally to benefit the patient (see Chapter 5).

The role and expected attributes of the modern general practitioner
have been summarized by a working party of the Welsh General Medical
Services Committee and the Welsh Council of the Royal College of
General Practitioners as follows:

By the year 2000 every general medical practitioner should have acquired
a respectful understanding of the complex determinants of health, illness
and disease with insight into the boundaries of professional knowledge.
The maintenance of well being and the restoration of health, by whatever means, depend in large measure on the body's own healing process,
influenced by genetic structure, nutrition, environmental factors, lifestyle, and sometimes assisted by intervention of a physical, psychological, social or spiritual nature.

The general practitioner recognizes the autonomy of all people and is
qualified and accredited to be responsible for personal, primary, continuing and preventive medical care delivered in ways appropriate to
individuals, families and small communities. The general practitioner
will normally attend patients near their homes in purpose-made, well
equipped premises or sometimes in a locality hospital. Home visits will
be a component of the general practitioner's work but reserved mainly
for the housebound. The cornerstone of the doctor's practice will be the
provision of integrated personal care sustained by the doctor – patient
relationship and a disciplined approach to every consultation.

Consultation with specialists (medical or social or professions allied
to medicine) will be at the general practitioner's discretion irrespective
of whether specialists consult in the centre, the local hospital or other
location.

Diagnoses and management plans will be framed to embrace physical,
psychological and contextual factors. A background understanding of
the determinants of health and the risks and benefits associated with
medical diagnostic, therapeutic or preventive interventions will be
essential. The general practitioner will also be skilled in helping people
to make appropriate personal choices of clinical interventions or of
problem-solving and decision-making processes in a local context. All
general practitioners will need protected time and support for continuing
education, audit or research.

The general practitioner and the associated core primary care team
(PHCT) will be expected to intervene educationally, preventively and
therapeutically to promote the patient's health.

A proportion of general practitioners will opt for further professional
training to prepare them for management positions as clinical directors
of fund holding practices or other health management roles. Those who
adopt such management roles must demonstrate a continuing involvement with the primary clinical services they purport to manage. Some

general practitioners from both groups will undergo a formal training in research and teaching that will prepare them for university appointments and academic leadership roles (Royal College of General Practitioners, 1996).

The differing clinical tasks in the two settings

It is clear that those patients who do reach hospital tend to have the rarer, more often life-threatening diseases, or atypical versions of the commoner ones. The hospital specialist is also presented with more developed and usually more organized diseases, which consequently can be more readily recognized. Indeed, diagnostic labels are likely to have been already attached by the general practitioner and may be known by the patient. Hospital doctors are also more likely to be presented with more clear-cut disease entities; for example, a patient who originally presented to his general practitioner with co-existing symptoms of both depression and diabetes is likely, on referral to a hospital diabetic clinic, to mention only the symptoms of thirst, polyuria and polydypsia. The other symptoms of early morning wakening and weepy spells will not be mentioned, since the general practitioner will have helped the patient to understand the nature of his symptoms and to differentiate one set of symptoms from the other. The patient is also likely to realize that the diabetic physician does not normally deal with depression.

Because of these factors, the hospital doctor can often make assumptions about the likely nature of the patient's presenting problems. For example, since a neurologist does not expect to encounter gynaecological problems they will not feature prominently in his clinical problem-solving. Furthermore, in the hospital setting confirmatory physical signs are more likely to be present and diagnostic problems are more likely to be exhaustively investigated, partly because of their potential severity and partly because of lack of continuing access to the patient. A specialty-specific routine work-up is also accorded to virtually all patients, irrespective of presenting features. In short, the hospital doctor tends to be over-inclusive although specialty-orientated.

The general practitioner, on the other hand, needs to develop skills as a primary assessor of problems. In a situation where patients have direct access, multiple problems are often presented in a single consultation, there are many symptoms but few clinical signs, and there is frequently a complex mix of physical, psychological and social factors, the general practitioner can make few prior suppositions concerning the likely nature of the presenting problems. They may be gynaecological and/or neurological and/or psychiatric, etc. Indeed, it is often not possible to identify a specific diagnosis. Furthermore, since many problems are presented early and in undifferentiated forms, it is frequently very difficult to predict their future course of development, let alone their likely outcome. Consequently, the general practitioner needs to be patient-oriented and has to develop the ability to be appropriately selective in history taking, performing physical examinations and the use of investigative facilities. General practitioners also have to be prepared to tolerate a greater degree of uncertainty because of the frequency with which they need to use time in both diagnosis and management. These themes will be further developed in Chapters 2–4.

Finally, whether practising in hospital or general practice, readers should always bear in mind the recent advice of the President of the General Medical Council regarding the expectations patients have of doctors:

> For patients, some old fashioned values and habits are still extremely important. In particular, they like seeing someone they know, someone whose performance as a doctor has given them confidence, someone who is easily accessible, and who will have taken the time and trouble to listen to their problems (Irvine, 1998).

Key points

- General practice is the level of care that lies between self- and hospital-care.
- Although patient illness behaviour is influenced by a large number of factors, the decision to consult a general practitioner is governed more by cultural and psychological factors than by physical symptoms of disease.
- The doctor must try to discover the particular reason or reasons for each patient's decision to consult.
- The symptoms patients present to their general practitioner tend to be 'unorganized' and undifferentiated, while those encountered in hospital tend to be 'medicalized' and more differentiated.
- The range, type, severity and frequency of problems encountered in general practice are very different from those encountered in hospital.
- In making clinical judgements about likely diagnoses and appropriate management plans, account must be taken of the particular context of the clinical task and its associated probabilities.
- Whatever the clinical context, clinicians must master both scientific *and* humanitarian aspects of the practice of medicine.

References

Armstrong, D. (1991). What do patients want? *British Medical Journal*, 303, 261.
Banks, M. H., Beresford S. A. A., Morrell D. C., Waller J. J. and Watkins C. J. (1975). Factors influencing demand for primary medical care in women aged 20–44 years: a preliminary report. *International Journal of Epidemiology*, 4, 189.
Barber, G. O. (1956). Medical education and the general practitioner. *Practitioner*, 176, 66.

Becker, M. H. (1979). Psychological aspects of health-related behaviour. In *Handbook of Medical Sociology* (H. Freeman, S. Levine and L. G. Reader, eds), 3rd edn. Englewood Cliffs, N.J.: Prentice Hall.

Bennett, J. R. and Atkinson, M. (1966). The differentiation between oesophageal and cardiac pain. *Lancet*, **2**, 1123.

Bentsen, B. G. (1976). The accuracy of recording patient problems in family practice. *Journal of Medical Education*, **51**, 311.

Davis, R. H. (1975). *General Practice for Students of Medicine*. London: Academic Press.

Dunnell, K and Cartwright, A. (1972). *Medicine Takers, Prescribers and Hoarders*. London: Routledge and MTP Press.

Federman, D. D. (1990). The education of medical students: sounds, alarums and excursions. *Academic Medicine*, **65**(4), 221–6.

Frank, P. I. (1970). Anterior chest pain in family practice. MD thesis, University of Liverpool.

Fry, J. (1993). *General Practice – the Facts*. Oxford: Radcliffe Medical Press.

Fry, J. and Sandler, G. (1993). *Common Diseases*, 5th edn. London: Kluwer Academic Publishers.

Gulbrandsen, P., Fugelli, P., Sandvik, L. and Hjortdahl, P. (1998). Influence of social problems on management in general practice: multipractice questionnaire survey. *British Medical Journal*, **317**, 28–32.

Hodgkin, K. (1978). *Towards Earlier Diagnosis in Primary Care*, 4th edn. Edinburgh: Churchill Livingstone.

Irvine, D. (1998). Foreword. In *GP Tomorrow* (J. Harrison and T. van Zwanenberg, eds.). Abingdon: Radcliffe Medical Press.

Jaco, G. E. (ed.) (1958). *Patients, Physicians and Illness: Sourcebook In Behavioural Science And Medicine*. New York: The Free Press.

Kohn, R. and White, K. L. (eds.) (1976). *Health care: an International Study*. Oxford: Oxford University Press.

Koos, E. L. (1954). *The Health of Regionville, What the People Thought and Did About It*. New York: Columbia University Press.

Lydeard, S. and Jones, R. (1989). Factors affecting the decision to consult with dyspepsia: comparison of consulters and non-consulters. *Journal of the Royal College of General Practitioners*, **39**, 495.

MacNaughton, J. (1998). Medicine and the arts: let's not forget the medicine. *British Journal of General Practice*, **48**, 952–3.

McWhinney, I. R. (1975). Family medicine in perspective. *New England Journal of Medicine*, **293**, 176.

Mechanic, D. (1961). The concept of illness behaviour. *Journal of Chronic Diseases*, **15**, 189.

Morrell, D. C. (1976). *An Introduction to Primary Medical Care*. Edinburgh: Churchill Livingstone.

Rashid, A. and Jagger, C. (1996). Patients' knowledge of anatomical location of major organs within the human body: a comparison between Asians and non-Asians. *Family Practice*, **13**, 450–54.

Rigge, M. (1998). What patients expect. In *GP Tomorrow* (J. Harrison and T. van Zwanenberg, eds.). Abingdon: Radcliffe Medical Press.

Ritchie, J., Jacoby, A. and Bone M. (1981). *Access To Primary Health Care*. London: HMSO.

Robinson, D. (1971). *The Process of Becoming Ill*. London: Routledge and Kegan Paul.

Royal College of General Practitioners (1996). *The Nature of General Medical Practice*. Report from General Practice 17. London: The Royal College of General Practitioners.

Starfield, B. (1992). *Primary Care: Concept, Evaluation and Policy*. New York: Oxford University Press.

Tarlov, A. R. (1988). In *The Task of Medicine* (K. L. White, ed.), p. ix. Menlo Park, California: The Henry J. Kaiser Family Foundation.

Walker, R. D. (1982) Knowledge of symptoms suggesting malignant disease amongst general practice patients. *Journal of the Royal College of General Practitioners*, **32**, 163.

Wilkin, D., Hallam, L., Leavey, R. and Metcalfe D. (1987a) *Anatomy of Urban General Practice*, pp. 81–105. London: Tavistock Publications.

Wilkin, D., Hallam, L., Leavey, R. and Metcalfe D. (1987b). *Anatomy of Urban General Practice*, pp. 106–135. London: Tavistock Publications.

Zola, I. K. (1973). Pathways to the doctor – from person to patient. *Social Science and Medicine*, 7, 677.

2

The consultation

Robin C. Fraser

No other human experience duplicates the
intimacy, candour, physical access and
vulnerability of seeing a doctor (Federman,
1990).

The consultation has been described as 'the essential unit of medical
practice' (Spence, 1960), and this is true whether it is conducted in
general practice or in hospital. If a clinician is deficient in essential
consultation competences, any other skills possessed become almost
irrelevant. Consequently, I would encourage the reader to focus heavily
on developing the ability to perform satisfactorily in consultation with
patients, since ' . . . all else in the practice of medicine derives from it'
(Spence, 1960).

   This chapter will provide an introduction to the tasks of the consultation
and then consider the necessary skills and competences which doctors need
to acquire in order to fulfil these tasks. It is hoped that this will enable
the reader to understand better the role of the consultation in clinical
practice and to develop a systematic approach to clinical behaviour within
the consultation, both of which should contribute to the development of
increased clinical competence. Although the chapter will focus on the
particular tasks and competences associated with consultations in general
practice, it will readily be recognized that most of these are also relevant to
consultations in hospital. Subsequent chapters in this book will expand
on particular aspects of the tasks and competences first outlined in this
chapter. In particular, Chapter 11 contains practical advice on how to
analyse and improve your consultation performance.

The tasks of the consultation

Stott and Davis (1979) have identified four broad tasks of the
consultation:

1. Identification and management of presenting problems
2. Management of continuing problems
3. Opportunistic anticipatory care
4. Modification of the patient's help-seeking behaviour.

It is important to appreciate that it may not be appropriate or possible to attempt all the potential tasks of the consultation on every occasion. Nevertheless, the consultation framework suggested by Stott and Davis provides a useful *aide-memoire* to action. In addition, Pendleton *et al.* (1984) have identified some of the more detailed component tasks of the consultation, and reference will be made to these in considering the four broad tasks in turn.

Task 1: Identification and management of presenting problems

This is the central task in almost every consultation. The normal sequence is for the doctor to attempt to identify what the presenting problems are, before considering an appropriate management plan. In identifying the presenting problem, the doctor will need to establish the reason(s) for the patient's attendance. This stage should encompass recognizing the nature of the problem and its effect on the patient, an elicitation of the patient's ideas, concerns and expectations, and an answer to the question: Why did the patient consult now? In identifying an appropriate management plan, the doctor should attempt to reach a shared understanding of the problem with the patient and be prepared to negotiate the details of management, while encouraging the patient to accept appropriate responsibility for carrying out all aspects of the agreed management plan.

It has been demonstrated that:

> By making patients part of the process of making decisions, the doctor becomes clearer about the nature of the patient's problem and the patient is more committed to any advice given. The result is a more satisfied patient, who will be more likely to follow medical advice (Savage and Armstrong, 1990).

One suggested way of 'making patients part of the process' is to encourage them to bring written lists of problems to the consultation (Middleton, 1995). Use of a patient's agenda form is associated, however, with the identification of more problems and with a tendency for reduced time to be allocated to individual problems (J. F. Middleton, personal communication).

The identification and management of presenting problems is the most traditional and predictable task of the consultation, which both general practitioners and hospital doctors would equally recognize. It has been suggested, however, that the following three tasks should also be considered if 'the exceptional potential in each primary care consultation is to be realized' (Stott and Davis, 1979).

Task 2: Management of continuing problems

As generalists who provide continuing care, doctors should not limit themselves to Task 1 (the identification and management of presenting problems), but should be prepared to extend the scope of the consultation to problems that they are aware patients have, even though patients have not requested them to do so. For example, if a patient attends with a sore throat, the doctor should be alert to the possible need to review the extent to which any co-existing diabetes/epilepsy/hypertension, etc., is under control. Such an unsolicited demonstration of interest by the doctor is again likely to result in higher levels of compliance with professional advice by the patient.

Task 3: Opportunistic anticipatory care

According to Stott and Davis (1979), 'One of the most exciting and controversial components of every consultation is the opportunity it provides for both the promotion of healthy lifestyles and early or presymptomatic diagnosis'. Although patients are usually quite happy for doctors to take such initiatives, it is essential that doctors do not become overzealous to the extent that they become insensitive to the true needs or wants of patients (Stott and Pill, 1990). Indeed, making 'repeated ritualistic interventions' through the provision of 'action oriented advice for those who are not ready to change is at best unhelpful, and could even entrench unhealthy behaviour' (Butler et al., 1998).

Task 4: Modification of the patient's help-seeking behaviour

It should be emphasized that the clinician's role in influencing the patient's future pattern of illness behaviour 'embodies both inappropriate under-use of medical services and their over-use' (Stott and Davis, 1979). Doctors should be able to enlighten their patients as to the circumstances when it would, or would not, be advantageous for them to seek medical care or to continue under medical supervision. This is a task of which undergraduates should be aware, but it is probably more appropriate that the necessary skills in patient education should be acquired and implemented at the postgraduate stage.

Consultation Tasks 1, 2 and 4 will be considered in detail in Chapters 3–6, while Task 3 will be dealt with in Chapters 7 and 8. Chapters 9–11 are relevant for all four consultation tasks.

The required consultation skills and competences

To be able to cope with the varied consultation tasks identified above and the associated challenges presented by patients, the clinician needs to master a broad range of skills. These include interpersonal skills (the ability to communicate and to make relationships with patients), reasoning skills (the ability to gather appropriate information, interpret and then apply it both in diagnosis and management) and practical skills (the ability to perform physical examinations and to use medical instruments).

Although there are many ways of analysing the professional capabilities that a doctor needs to possess in the consultation, the following seven major categories of consultation competence and 35 component competences (as contained in the Leicester Assessment Package) have been shown to be valid and acceptable in the setting of general practice (Fraser *et al.*, 1994). With minor modifications, they have also been shown to be valid and acceptable for undergraduate teaching and assessment purposes in a hospital context (Hastings *et al.*, in press; McKinley *et al.*, in press).

Categories of consultation competence (and relative weightings)

1. Interviewing/history-taking (20%)
2. Physical examination (10%)
3. Patient management (20%)
4. Problem-solving (20%)
5. Behaviour/relationship with patients (10%)
6. Anticipatory care (10%)
7. Record-keeping (10%).

The percentages represent the relative degree of importance of the various categories, and these have been derived from a mixture of published evidence and professional consensus (see Fraser *et al.*, 1994). The most important – and the most difficult to acquire – are competence in interviewing/history taking, patient management and problem-solving. The category concerning record-keeping is the least important for undergraduates.

Within each of these seven broad categories are a number of component competences (see below). Inevitably, some overlap occurs between components of different categories. It will not, of course, be necessary or appropriate for a doctor to employ every one of these listed competences in every consultation. Some will be required in every consultation (for example, the need to listen attentively, the need to maintain a friendly but professional relationship, etc.), but others will be required only in a minority of consultations (for example, use of investigations, referrals to hospital, opportunistic health promotion). Much will depend on the nature of the clinical challenge(s) faced by the doctor in any particular consultation.

Detailed component consultation competences

Interviewing/history-taking

- Introduces self to patients
- Puts patients at ease

- Allows patients to elaborate presenting problem fully
- Listens attentively
- Seeks clarification of words used by patients as appropriate
- Phrases questions simply and clearly
- Uses silence appropriately
- Recognizes patients' verbal and non-verbal cues
- Identifies patients' reasons for consultation
- Elicits relevant and specific information from patients and/or their records to help distinguish between working diagnoses
- Considers physical, social and psychological factors as appropriate
- Exhibits well-organized approach to information gathering.
  (See Chapters 3 and 6 in particular.)

Physical examination

- Performs examination and elicits physical signs correctly and sensitively
- Uses the instruments commonly used in general practice in a selective, competent and sensitive manner.

Patient management

- Formulates management plans appropriate to findings and circumstances in collaboration with patients
- Makes discriminating use of investigations, referral and drug therapy
- Is prepared to use time appropriately
- Demonstrates understanding of the importance of reassurance and explanation and uses clear and understandable language
- Checks patients' level of understanding
- Arranges appropriate follow-up
- Attempts to modify help-seeking behaviour of patients as appropriate.
  (See Chapter 4 in particular.)

Problem-solving

- Generates appropriate working diagnoses or identifies problems depending on circumstances
- Seeks relevant and discriminating physical signs to help confirm or refute working diagnoses
- Correctly interprets and applies information obtained from patient records, history, physical examination and investigations
- Is capable of applying knowledge of basic, behavioural and clinical sciences to the identification, management and solution of patients' problems
- Recognizes limits of competence and responds appropriately.
  (See Chapters 3 and 4 in particular.)

Behaviour/relationship with patients

- Maintains friendly but professional relationship with patients with due regard to the ethics of medical practice
- Conveys sensitivity to the needs of patients
- Demonstrates an awareness that the patient's attitude to the doctor (and vice versa) affects management and achievement of levels of co-operation and compliance.
  (See Chapters 5 and 9 in particular.)

Anticipatory care

- Acts on appropriate opportunities for health promotion and disease prevention
- Provides sufficient explanation to patients for preventive initiatives taken
- Sensitively attempts to enlist the co-operation of patients to promote change to healthier lifestyles.
  (See Chapters 7 and 8 in particular.)

Record-keeping

- Makes accurate, legible and appropriate records of every doctor–patient contact and referral
- The minimum information recorded should include date of consultation, relevant history and examination findings, any measurement carried out (e.g. blood pressure, peak flow, weight, etc.), the diagnosis or problem (preferably 'boxed'), outline of management plan, investigations ordered and follow-up arrangements
- If a prescription is issued, the names of drugs, dose, quantity provided and special precautions intimated to the patient should be recorded.

It should be noted that the category 'Physical examination' relates to technical and manipulative skills *only*; the cognitive skill of deciding *what* to examine is covered under the category of 'Problem-solving' ('seeks relevant and discriminating physical signs to help confirm or refute working diagnoses'). It should also be noted that preventive aspects relating to the management of presenting problems should be covered under the category 'Patient management', whereas the category 'Anticipatory care' relates to opportunistic preventive interventions unrelated to the patient's presenting complaint(s).

Evidence-based consultations

In all three editions of this book the authors have made every attempt to provide 'corroborative evidence for their stated views' on various aspects of clinical method and practice (Fraser, 1987). More recently the concept of evidence-based practice has become more explicit, and an increasingly influential evidence-based medicine movement has grown up (Evidence-based Medicine Working Group, 1992). Evidence-based medicine has been defined as:

> the conscientious, explicit and judicious use of current best evidence in making decisions about the care of individual patients (Sackett *et al.*, 1996).

The general view is that the evidence-based medicine movement has 'done a good job in focusing explicit attention on the application of evidence from valid clinical research to clinical practice' (Knottnerus and Dinant, 1997).

Furthermore, there is a growing awareness – and acceptance – that 'clinical decisions . . . can no longer be comfortably based on opinion alone', and that 'accessing and appraising evidence is rapidly becoming a core clinical competency' in itself (Scully and Donaldson, 1998). Clinicians are faced with many potential problems, however, in accessing and implementing the results of research findings in everyday clinical practice (Sheldon *et al.*, 1998). Detailed consideration of these difficulties is beyond the scope of this book, but the main factors are '. . . the quality of the research, the degree of uncertainty of the findings, relevance to the clinical setting, whether the benefits to the patient outweigh any adverse effects, and whether the overall benefits justify the costs when competing priorities and available resources are taken into account' (Sheldon *et al.*, 1998). It also needs to be acknowledged that in many consultations – especially in primary care – no conclusive evidence is available on which to base decisions.

Nevertheless, clinicians should always strive to 'base their personal practice, wherever possible, on objective research evidence of best practice, even when this conflicts with their past or current professional habits' (Fraser *et al.*, 1998). It should be evident to the reader that this state of mind underpins many, if not most, of the consultation competences outlined earlier in this chapter. However, when definitive evidence is absent or incomplete, patients must then rely on the capacity of clinicians to make sound professional judgements.

Patient-centred consultations

Over the past 50 years or so, substantial changes have occurred in the expectations of, and interactions between, doctors and patients in the consultation (Armstrong, 1991). Previously, consultations were rather doctor-centred as many doctors tended to be authoritarian, paternalistic and domineering. The scope of the consultation was frequently limited to consideration of the patient's physical symptoms and signs only. Patients tended to be rather passive, relying almost totally on the doctor's judgement, and only rarely would they call upon doctors to justify their decisions and actions.

That situation has been transformed. There is now a greater recognition, by both doctors and patients, that the consultation should be more of a dialogue. Indeed the consultation has been described as 'a meeting between experts' (Tuckett et al., 1985), since patients can be regarded as experts on their bodily feelings and their understanding of them. It has in fact been demonstrated that patients can develop elaborate and often sophisticated theories concerning their own illness (Tuckett et al., 1985) to which doctors should pay attention.

As consultations have become much more patient-centred, doctors have permitted, and even encouraged, patients to report not only their symptoms but also their thoughts and feelings about their illness and their expectations of the consultation. Thus, doctors and patients have broadened the scope of the consultation through 'a shift from thinking about patient care in terms of disease and pathology towards thinking in terms of people and their problems' (Henbest and Stewart, 1990). Furthermore, there is a growing awareness that 'patients' wants are not capricious whims but needs in themselves' and that what patients value most of all in the consultation is 'a doctor who listens' (Armstrong, 1991).

This major shift in the style and scope of consultations in general practice is vividly described by an anonymous ex-surgeon who became a family practitioner:

> I am available to take care of diseases but that's not all I do. My patients are much larger than their diseases. Now I feel that I am really doing something for patients – that there is really something to practising medicine. The best thing we can do for patients is to understand what they say, and a prerequisite is listening. Obviously I take care of their diseases – I am available to do that in ways that they need me – but that's a small part of what I do (Dr. C, in Starfield, 1992).

Patient-centred consultations and health outcomes

To what extent does a patient-centred approach have any effect on the patient's state of health? Following an extensive review of the literature, Horder and Moore (1990) concluded that, in addition to the fulfilment of the necessary technical tasks of the consultation (i.e. history-taking and therapeutic management), interpersonal or socio-emotional aspects of the consultation play a major role in influencing health outcomes. The results of a number of experimental studies involving intervention and control groups suggested that there was a relationship between the way in which doctors and patients behave during a consultation and the patients' subsequent state of health (Kaplan *et al.*, 1989). In particular,

> more control by patients, more expression of emotion (positive or negative) by either patient or doctor and more information sought by patients and given by the doctor, were associated with better health on follow-up, especially as revealed in functional capacity and physiological measurements (Horder and Moore, 1990).

These beneficial effects were demonstrated in separate studies involving patients with the diverse conditions of diabetes mellitus, hypertension and peptic ulcer. For example, those diabetic patients exposed to a more patient-centred approach achieved better control of their diabetes, as evidenced by significantly better levels of glycosylated haemoglobin, compared to a control group.

Furthermore, it has been established that hypertensive patients of doctors who received a 2-hour tutorial concentrating on reasons for failure in controlling blood pressure, barriers to compliance and patients' needs for knowledge achieved a significant improvement in the control of raised blood pressure compared to a control group of patients whose doctors had not had such a tutorial (Inui *et al.*, 1976). The underlying strategy for altering compliance was to stress to the doctors the need to study the patients' own ideas about hypertension and its treatment. The authors concluded:

> . . . studying patient beliefs and influencing them proved to be more important elements in the consultation than the review of symptoms or the physical examination . . . . Helping patients to learn and understand resulted in better control of blood pressure through better compliance.

Further supporting evidence is available from the findings of two studies carried out in Canadian general practice. In a study of the natural history of headache, the most important factor in predicting recovery was that the patients concerned 'had had good opportunity to discuss their problems with the doctor' (Bass *et al.*, 1986a). In a further study of patients presenting to their doctor with new symptoms it was established that 'the factor most strongly associated with recovery at 1 month was the patient's complete agreement with the doctor's opinion' (Bass *et al.*, 1986b).

It seems, therefore, that a patient-centred approach really does make a difference. It does not mean, however, that doctors can neglect the traditional consultation skills of history taking, physical examination and therapeutic management. It does mean that doctors need to incorporate these into an overall patient-centred consultation style. Finally, the reader should be aware of the following warning as to the reasons for unsatisfactory consultations:

Bad consultations result from having insufficient clinical knowledge, from failing to relate to patients or from failing to understand the patient's behaviour, his perception of his illness or its context (Howie, 1985).

Key points

- The consultation between doctor and patient is the fundamental event in clinical practice, whether in general practice or hospital.
- To become clinically competent a doctor needs to acquire a broad range of interpersonal, reasoning and practical skills.
- Whenever possible doctors should base their consulting behaviour on research evidence of best practice, even when this conflicts with their usual professional habits.
- The primary task of the consultation is to establish the reason(s) for the patient's attendance.
- A patient-centred consultation approach results in significantly improved health outcomes for patients.
- The exceptional potential of every consultation in general practice needs to be recognized and appropriately acted upon.

References

Armstrong, D. (1991). What do patients want? *British Medical Journal*, 303, 261.

Bass, M. J., McWhinney, I. R., Dempsey, I. B. *et al.* (1986a). Predictors of outcome in headache patients presenting to family practitioners – a one year prospective study. *Headache Journal*, 26(6), 285.

Bass, M. J., Buck, C., Turner, L. *et al.* (1986b). The physician's actions and the outcome of illness. *Journal of Family Practice*, 23, 43.

Butler, C. C., Pill, R. and Stott, N. C. H. (1998). Qualitative study of patients' perceptions of doctors' advice to quit smoking: implications for opportunistic health promotion. *British Medical Journal*, 316, 1878–81.

Dr C. (1992). First contact care and gatekeepers. In *Primary Care: Concept, Evaluation and Policy*. New York: Oxford University Press.

Evidence-based Medicine Working Group (1992). Evidence-based medicine: a new approach to teaching the practice of medicine. *Journal of the American Medical Academy*, 268, 420–25.

Federman, D. D. (1990). The education of medical students: sounds, alarms and excursions. *Academic Medicine*, 65(4), 221–6.

Fraser, R. C. (1987). Preface to the first edition. In *Clinical Method: A General Practice Approach* (R. C. Fraser, ed.). Oxford: Butterworth-Heinemann.

Fraser, R. C., McKinley, R. K. and Mulholland, H. (1994). Consultation competence in general practice: establishing the face validity of prioritized criteria in the Leicester Assessment Package. *British Journal of General Practice*, 44, 109–13.

Fraser. R. C., Baker, R. and Lakhani M. K. (1998). Evidence-based clinical audit: an overview. In *Evidence-based Audit in General Practice: From Principles to Practice* (R. C. Fraser, M. K. Lakhani and R. H. Baker, eds.), pp. 1–15. Oxford: Butterworth-Heinemann.

Hastings. A. M., Fraser. R. C., and McKinley. R. K. (in press). A new integrated course in clinical methods for medical students.

Henbest, R. J. and Stewart, M. (1990). Patient-centredness in the consultation. II: Does it really make a difference? *Family Practice*, 7, 28.

Horder. J. and Moore, G. T. (1990). The consultation and health outcomes (editorial). *British Journal of General Practice*, 40, 442.

Howie, J. G. R. (1985). The consultation: a multipurpose framework. In *Decision Making in General Practice* (M. Sheldon, J. Brooke and A. Rector, eds.) Basingstoke: Macmillan.

Inui. T. S., Yourtree. E. L. and Williamson I. W. (1976). Improved outcomes in hypertension after physician tutorials. A controlled trial. *Annals of Internal Medicine*, 84, 646.

Kaplan. S. H., Greenfield. S. and Ware, J. F. (1989). Assessing the effects of patient–physician interactions on the outcomes of chronic disease. *Medical Care*, 27, 110.

Knottnerus, J. A. and Dinant, G. J. (1997). Medicine-based evidence, a prerequisite for evidence-based medicine. *British Medical Journal*, 315, 1109–10.

McKinley. R. K., Fraser. R. C., van der Vleuten, C. and Hastings, A. M. (in press). Formative assessment of the consultation performance of medical students in the setting of general practice using a modified version of the Leicester Assessment Package.

Middleton, J. F. (1995). Asking the patient to bring a list: a feasibility study. *British Medical Journal*, 311, 34.

Pendleton, D., Schofield, T., Tate, P. and Havelock, P. (1984). *The Consultation: An Approach to Learning and Teaching*. Oxford: Oxford University Press.

Sackett, D. L., Rosenberg, W. M. C., Gray, J. A. M. *et al.* (1996). Evidence-based medicine: what it is and what it isn't. It's about integrating individual clinical expertise and the best external evidence. *British Medical Journal*, 312, 71–2.

Savage, R. and Armstrong, D. (1990). Effect of a general practitioner's consulting style on patients' satisfaction: a controlled study. *British Medical Journal*, 301, 1968.

Scully, G. and Donaldson, L. J. (1998). Clinical governance and the drive for quality improvement in the new NHS in England. *British Medical Journal*, 317, 62–5.

Sheldon, T. A., Guyatt, G. H. and Haines, A. (1998). Getting research findings into practice: when to act on the evidence. *British Medical Journal*, 317, 139–42.

Spence, J. (1960). The need for understanding the individual as part of the training and function of doctors and nurses. National Association for Mental Health. Reprinted in *The Purpose and Practice of Medicine*, pp. 271–80. Oxford: Oxford University Press.

Stott, N. C. H. and Davis, R. H. (1979). The exceptional potential in each primary care consultation. *Journal of the Royal College of General Practitioners*, 29, 201.

Stott, N. C. H. and Pill R. M. (1990). Advise yes, dictate no. Patients' views on health promotion in the consultation. *Family Practice*, 7, 125.

Tuckett. D., Boulton. M., Olson. C. and Williams, A. (1985). *Meetings between Experts: An Approach to sharing Ideas in Medical Consultations*. London: Tavistock Publications.

3
The diagnostic process
Robin C. Fraser

The ability to cope with uncertainty, exclude
the dangerous, ignore the irrelevant . . .
(Elwyn, 1997).

When patients present with new problems, attempting to arrive at a
diagnosis is perhaps the single most important consultation task for a
doctor, whether in hospital or general practice. If it is possible to make a
definitive diagnosis, the doctor becomes more aware not only of the
specific pathophysiology underlying a patient's complaint, but also of its
probable natural history. Such understanding greatly influences the way
in which plans for clinical management are formulated and implemented.
The greater the confidence the doctor has in any diagnosis made, the
greater is the ability to judge not only whether, but also what sort of,
intervention is indicated. Thus, arriving at a diagnosis 'is a crucial
achievement which opens the way to prognosis and treatment' (Royal
College of General Practitioners, 1972).

It must be emphasized, however, that the term 'diagnosis' does not just
refer to conventional disease labels; nor does the term 'pathophysiology'
refer solely to organic disease. Although the search for, and identification
of, organic disease (i.e. disease-centred diagnosis) is a crucially important
consultation task, it is not the whole story. It is also necessary to attempt
to arrive at a patient-centred diagnosis, i.e. one which includes consideration of the patient's thoughts and feelings concerning the nature
and potential causes of their presenting complaints (see previous
chapter). Thus, the reader is encouraged to consider diagnoses in whole-
person terms, which should include both patient-centred and disease-
centred elements.

In this regard, the reader should also be aware that making a firm
pathophysiological diagnosis in general practice may not be possible –
even for experienced doctors – in anything up to 50% of presenting
patients. In the absence of an appropriate diagnostic label, however, the
'diagnosis' can still be expressed in the form of the patient's problem(s)
(see also 'The triple diagnosis', below).

In this book, the diagnostic process and management are considered
in separate chapters for the sake of convenience and clarity. It should be

remembered, however, that a diagnosis is usually a statement of probability rather than certainty, and often needs to be 'regarded as provisional until supported by the subsequent course of the case or the response to specific treatment' (Royal College of General Practitioners, 1972). Thus, although diagnosis often precedes and predicts management plans and actions, the diagnostic process often includes management. This is because management decisions are frequently, and justifiably, taken on the basis of an assessment of the patient's symptoms and/or signs and/or problems, without a definitive diagnosis having been made. Although this happens in both general practice and hospital, it is especially frequent in the former.

Making a diagnosis is a complex process and involves far more than merely amassing clinical information. A wide range of skills needs to be acquired, integrated and applied (see Chapter 2). Of particular importance are skills in interviewing (see Chapter 6), clinical reasoning and accessing personal knowledge at the time when it is required. Thus:

> The term [diagnosis] encompasses those processes whereby the clinician interprets clinical information [and] follows and chooses among his thoughts about what is wrong with the patient (Gale and Marsden, 1985).

It is essential to develop the ability to arrive at a 'correct' diagnosis as often as clinical circumstances permit. If this goal is to be achieved, you will need first of all to develop the capability to understand how diagnoses are made and why in particular circumstances you have arrived at the correct diagnosis. You are then more likely to continue to arrive at correct diagnoses on future occasions. Since many, if not most, errors in diagnosis result from errors in the diagnostic process rather than from a lack of factual knowledge, you will also be better equipped to identify possible reasons for such errors and to take appropriate action to rectify the situation. Such a process of self-learning is a powerful stimulus to improvement in clinical performance as it will enable you to cope better when, as is inevitable, you are faced with clinical problems not previously encountered.

This chapter will introduce the reader to the processes by which problems are clarified and diagnoses are formulated.

Inductive and hypothetico-deductive methods of problem-solving

In the final resort, doctors arrive at a diagnosis when they are able to fit a patient's symptoms and signs into a pattern that they can recognize as representing a particular disease entity. In hospital practice there is a greater likelihood of being able to do this as compared to general practice.

Nevertheless, in any clinical context, only rarely is a distinctive pattern instantly recognizable; usually a doctor needs to embark on a search for further evidence to help to distinguish between a number of potential diagnoses. There are several ways in which this task can be accomplished. Often it can be done within a single consultation, but sometimes it requires more than one.

It is likely that you will have been taught to reach a diagnosis by using the traditional or inductive method of problem-solving (Figure 3.1). This method dictates that – irrespective of presenting complaint – a comprehensive history (including a system review) has to be taken from every patient, followed by a complete physical examination backed up by a number of investigations, many of which are of a routine nature. Furthermore, you will have been encouraged to delay the task of diagnostic formulation (i.e. interpreting the information gathered) until this mass of information has been assembled.

This approach undoubtedly provides medical students with repeated opportunities to familiarize themselves with the range of questions that may need to be asked in taking histories from patients, and gives them the necessary practice for developing their skills in physical examination techniques. In actual clinical practice, however, such an approach to clinical problem-solving is rarely used by general practitioners and infrequently by hospital doctors because 'an unfocused shotgun approach is unproductive, confusing and time-consuming' (Joorabchi, 1989).

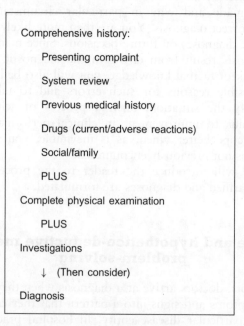

Comprehensive history:

　　Presenting complaint

　　System review

　　Previous medical history

　　Drugs (current/adverse reactions)

　　Social/family

PLUS

Complete physical examination

PLUS

Investigations

　　↓　(Then consider)

Diagnosis

Figure 3.1　Inductive method of problem-solving

Indeed, 'excessive data collection interferes with clinical inference and reasoning by overloading the capacity of the system (i.e. the doctor)' (Hoffbrand, 1989). Consequently, the inductive approach should be reserved for the few occasions when patients present with such vague symptoms that no useful diagnostic formulations can be generated and potentially serious underlying causes cannot be excluded.

In reality, most clinicians reach diagnoses by a process of hypothetico-deductive reasoning, i.e. by educated guessing and testing (Elstein *et al.*, 1978). Furthermore, studies have shown that general practitioners and hospital doctors both use the same 'multiple hypotheses-guided, problem orientated enquiry' (Barrows *et al.*, 1982). Figure 3.2 provides a simplified representation of the stages involved in this process. The so-called hypothetico-deductive method is efficient as it enables doctors to solve problems with maximum time- and cost-effectiveness and minimal disturbance to patients. A professor of medicine has given further support to this view: 'In recognizing that diagnosis is fundamentally hypothetico-deductive, I am not simply contrasting it with a blank mind ritualistically collecting information, I am saying it is superior because a blank mind may miss information which is generated only in response to an idea' (Campbell, 1987).

Even before a patient enters a consulting room, whether in hospital or general practice, a clinician is likely to have access to a considerable store of information about that patient. If the doctor knows the patient well – as is likely with a significant proportion of patients in general practice – knowledge of the patient's previous medical history, individual and family circumstances and previous patterns of illness behaviour may be readily recalled from memory.

If the patient is not known to the consulting clinician – as will be the case in the majority of consultations conducted by students – the medical record should always be selectively scrutinized *before* the patient enters the consulting room. With practice, this can be done in a matter of 10–20 seconds. The time invested will be repaid in the majority of consultations by arming the clinician with much valuable information, which will facilitate more efficient clinical problem-solving. The following information should be sought:

- Age, sex and social class; the latter can be gleaned from the patient's address and/or occupation. All these factors have an influence when considering diagnostic probabilities.
- Significant previous medical history/family history: the medical records in most (teaching) practices will have these conveniently summarized. This will help you to avoid asking needless questions (for example, if a patient has had a hysterectomy you need not ask about menstruation) or may assist in the erection of diagnostic hypotheses (for example, if a patient has had an appendicectomy then appendicitis cannot be the cause of any presentation of abdominal pain).

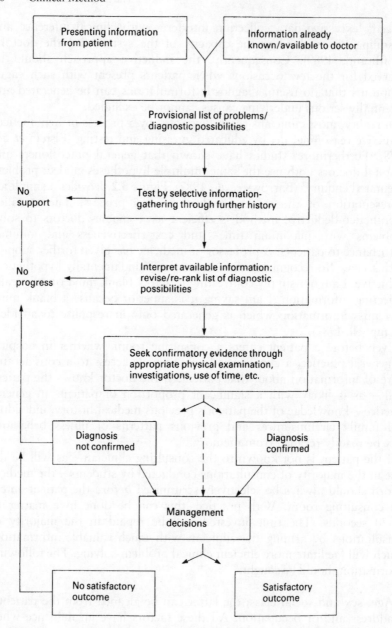

Figure 3.2 Hypothetico-deductive method of problem-solving (adapted from Elstein *et al.*, 1978)

Furthermore, knowledge of current medication may help you to link a patient's presenting symptoms with particular drug side-effects. An awareness that a patient's family member had previously died of cancer, heart disease, etc. may also alert you to the fact that the patient's presenting symptoms may relate to anxiety about having contracted the same disease.

- Frequency of attendance: this will provide some insight into the ability of the patient to tolerate symptoms. It is usually wise to pay particular attention to any presentations from infrequent attenders.
- Details of the last consultation: the reason(s) for the current consultation may well relate to the patient's last consultation. If so, this will often signify that the patient's symptoms will not have resolved as expected or else that new ones have developed. In any event, you will be aware of what took place previously and this will make your current consultation more efficient.

As the consultation begins, the doctor is presented with information that is both verbal and non-verbal. There is now considerable evidence to indicate that: 'experienced doctors often formulate their diagnostic hypotheses in the very first few instances with the patient and they are usually correct' (van der Vleuten, 1996). In many instances a prior stage of 'pre-diagnostic interpretation' (Gale and Marsden, 1983) occurs, during which the doctor begins to assess the patient's problems in terms of broad categorizations rather than specific diagnostic entities – e.g. 'I think the problem is cardiovascular'; 'this is likely to be psychological rather than physical', 'acute rather than chronic', 'serious rather than trivial', etc.

In the next phase of the problem-solving process, the doctor seeks to gather further information by asking particular questions of the patient in an attempt to find support for, and to discriminate between, the diagnostic possibilities previously generated. Throughout the process, the doctor needs to be constantly interpreting the answers received from the patient and modifying the search for further information accordingly. The immediate aim is to try to eliminate any previously nominated diagnostic possibility that is not supported by the additional information gathered. The ultimate aim is to be left with a single definitive diagnosis: more usually, however, the doctor will be left with one or more diagnostic probabilities.

Since the history is the key predictor of eventual diagnosis (see below), the purpose of the physical examination is to seek *relevant and discriminating* physical signs to help confirm or refute working diagnoses (Fraser, 1994; Sandler, 1984).

If at any stage in the problem-solving process no support can be gathered and no progress can be made, the presenting problem needs to be reconsidered and a fresh assessment of the likely diagnoses made through the gathering and interpretation of further clinical information. If a diagnosis is confirmed, management decisions can then be implemented as appropriate. On the other hand, a final judgement may have to be postponed because of insufficient evidence to confirm or eliminate a diagnostic possibility. Under these circumstances, a 'non-diagnosis' may have to be made or time employed as a deliberate diagnostic strategy. Thus, management decisions may have to be made in the absence of a firm diagnosis, and the outcome awaited. Particular aspects of this process will be considered in greater detail in due course.

The relative contribution of the clinical history, physical examination and investigations in the diagnostic process

Regrettably, the value of the history in the diagnosis of disease often seems to be neglected in both undergraduate and postgraduate medical education (Sandler, 1984).

Most of the clinical problems encountered in everyday clinical practice can be dealt with effectively and satisfactorily on the basis of a good clinical history (Sandler, 1984). Thus, history-taking is the key to diagnosis in the consultation. This is particularly true in general practice because of the many presentations of multiple, undifferentiated symptoms, often with a paucity of accompanying physical signs and the frequent absence of 'disease' (see Chapter 1). The results of two studies based on new referrals to outpatient departments of two hospitals in Nottingham and Barnsley confirm, perhaps more surprisingly, that it is also true in hospital practice.

Hampton et al. (1975) showed that the diagnosis can be made on the basis of the clinical history alone in 83% of new patients seen in a cardiology outpatient clinic, compared to physical examination (9%) and investigations (9%). In a more comprehensive study in a medical outpatient department, Sandler (1979) also concluded that the diagnostic value of the history far outweighed the contribution of physical examination or investigations. The history alone determined the diagnosis in 56% of all referrals made, with a range of 27–67% for alimentary and cardiovascular diagnoses respectively. Physical examination determined 17% of diagnoses, with a range of 0–24% (alimentary and cardiovascular, respectively). The corresponding figures for routine investigations were 5%, with a range of 0–17% (alimentary and respiratory, respectively) and for special investigations 18%, with a range of 6–58% (cardiovascular and alimentary, respectively). Routine haematological and urine examinations made a negligible (1%) contribution to diagnosis.

When the 180 patients with chest pain were considered separately, it is interesting to note that:

The history gave the diagnosis in 90%, and the examination was of no diagnostic value at all. Routine investigations, mainly chest radiographs and electrocardiography, helped with only 3% of diagnoses and special tests, mainly exercise electrocardiography, with 6% (Sandler, 1979).

Modern technology has made it all too easy to carry out batteries of tests. Consequently, there is 'frequently an unfortunate tendency to rely on the results of such tests before decisions are taken on diagnosis and treatment, even though such tests are often of limited value' (Sandler, 1984). This has been amply demonstrated above.

On the basis of these findings, Sandler concluded:

> *Much greater emphasis should be placed on the diagnostic . . . value of the history. Students, and postgraduates, should be well trained in taking a good history and in drawing diagnostic conclusions from the history before embarking on the examination. This will encourage the student to seek specific examination findings to confirm or refute the diagnosis based on the history* [my italics].

This is probably the most important statement contained in this book. If all doctors could acquire and implement the necessary skills, it would result in a major improvement in the quality and cost-effectiveness of clinical practice, not least through a reduction in the ordering of unnecessary tests and investigations. It would also improve the quality of medical education by providing more appropriate role models for medical students (and junior doctors) to emulate.

A Dean of Medicine emphasized the point:

> If you can take a good medical history, trust your physical examination and safely judge how sick your patient is, you can avoid excessive testing, imaging and prescribing (Federman, 1990).

It must be stressed, however, that 'a good history' must mean an appropriate and suitably discriminating history. 'This means asking the *right* question, not *every* question' (Hoffbrand, 1989) [my italics]. For example, thyrotoxicosis is a condition in which dozens of clinical features may occur. If thyrotoxicosis were suspected, it would make more sense for the doctor to try and establish whether the patient had weight loss with an increased appetite and dislike of hot weather, since the presence of these three features would make the diagnosis highly likely. On the other hand, symptoms like tiredness and irritability can occur in many other conditions apart from thyrotoxicosis and are, therefore, not key symptoms in helping to discriminate between thyrotoxicosis and other conditions (see Case 2 below). As Dixon (1986) has noted with impeccable logic, 'It makes no sense to ask a lot of history questions that will make no difference to the outcome of the consultation'.

The over-riding importance of the history in clinical medicine is further reinforced when one considers the major contribution it makes not only to diagnosis but also to determining management plans (see Chapter 4).

Generating and ranking appropriate diagnostic possibilities

There are four principal factors which influence the generation and ranking of diagnostic possibilities: probability, seriousness, treatability and novelty (Elstein *et al.*, 1971).

Probability

This is by far the most important influence since, in any given clinical circumstance, the essential question a doctor must ask is: What is the most likely cause or causes of my patient's symptoms? The probability that a particular presenting symptom or group of symptoms will result in a particular diagnosis being made is further influenced by two inter-related factors:

- The crude frequency of occurrence of the particular condition(s) suspected
- The complex interaction of patient and symptom variables and its effect on that crude frequency.

As an example, consider the presenting symptom of cough. Our knowledge of the distribution of morbidity within general practice tells us that the overwhelming likelihood is that the cough is caused by an acute infection of non-serious nature (see Table 1.11). Furthermore, consider the way that diagnostic probabilities will be influenced both by variations in the duration of the cough and the age of the particular patient (Figures 3.3 and 3.4, respectively). It is obvious that the likely diagnosis is very different for a 3-year-old with a cough – whatever its duration – compared to a 70-year-old. Likewise, the probable diagnosis of a cough in a 70-year-old will greatly vary depending on whether it has been present for 3 days or 3 months. On the basis of an awareness of probabilities, therefore, a doctor is immediately helped towards the appropriate interpretation of a patient's presenting symptom even at this early stage of the consultation. The elicitation of the presence or absence of associated symptoms such as haemoptysis, weight loss, etc., will of course further influence and help to clarify the diagnostic probabilities.

It is important to remember, however, that the most likely underlying diagnosis need not always be of a non-serious nature. For example, if a man of 50 presents with severe crushing and central chest pain radiating into both his jaw and his left arm, accompanied by dyspnoea and sweating, the most likely diagnosis is myocardial infarction. Indeed, with such a clinical picture any other diagnosis is unlikely.

Seriousness

Particular consideration should be given to the possibility that a life-threatening or seriously incapacitating condition may be responsible for

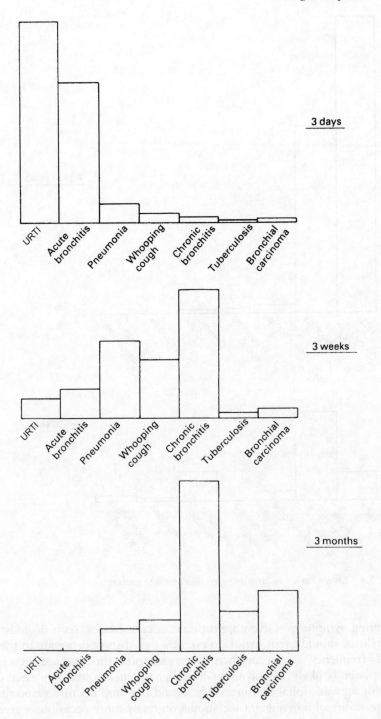

Figure 3.3   Likelihood of different causes of cough relative to duration of symptom

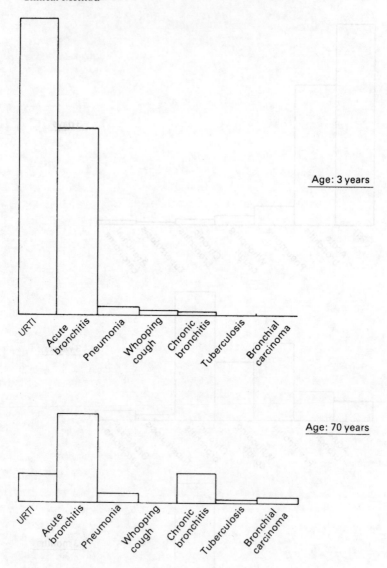

Figure 3.4   Likely causes of cough in two different age groups

presenting symptoms. Given appropriate circumstances, such diagnostic possibilities should merit inclusion even though disproportionate to their actual frequency of occurrence. For example, the average general practitioner is likely to encounter a malignant melanoma only once or twice in a professional lifetime. This should not stop doctors suspecting the possibility of a malignant melanoma on many more occasions – given an appropriate clinical presentation – because of the potentially catastrophic consequences of delay in making such a diagnosis.

Treatability

The more amenable to treatment a potential underlying cause for presenting symptoms is, the more likely it is to be included as a diagnostic possibility and the higher its ranking is likely to be. For example, myxoedema is an uncommon cause of tiredness but should not be overlooked as it is readily corrected by replacement therapy.

Novelty

Very rare, but memorable, conditions are disproportionately likely to be included in a potential list of causes. For example, students frequently suggest phaeochromocytoma as a diagnostic probability, although there would be little likelihood of encountering a single case in a professional lifetime in general practice. The temptation to include such diagnoses should be resisted!

Novelty diagnoses are particularly likely to be suggested if the individual doctor (or student) concerned has had recent personal experience of a dramatic or tragic event (Slovic et al., 1982). For example, missing the diagnosis of temporal arteritis, resulting in blindness for the unfortunate patient, is likely to lead to subsequent over-diagnosis of such a condition.

When faced with the practical problem of generating appropriate differential diagnoses, you should aim to produce a list with *two distinct categories*. The first should contain the *most likely* causes and initially include a maximum of five possibilities. The second should encompass the *less likely but important to consider* possibilities, encompassing the serious and treatable categories. This should consist of one or two possibilities only. These particular numerical limits are recommended because formal research studies indicate that the capacity of a doctor's mind to retain complex items in the memory – such as diagnostic hypotheses – has a limit of seven (Campbell, 1987). Novelty contributions should feature rarely.

Difficulties students experience in making diagnoses

Whatever the method of problem-solving used, there are two principal reasons why medical students are likely to experience particular difficulty – at least initially – in arriving at appropriate diagnoses in the setting of general practice.

The first reason relates to the particular nature of general practice and the student's unfamiliarity with it. This topic has been fully dealt with in Chapter 1, which highlighted the differences in diagnostic probabilities between hospital and general practice settings. Furthermore, because of the essential differences in the types of problems presented, there is a decreased likelihood in absolute terms of being able to make definitive diagnoses in general practice as compared to hospital. This can be a source of both frustration and confusion. In addition, you will need to come to terms with the reality that general practitioners 'must often diagnose what things are not, rather than what they are' (Dixon, 1986). For example, the doctor may have to say to a patient with abdominal pain who is not ill, 'I don't know what is causing your pain but I'm sure it's nothing serious and in particular I can reassure you that it's not appendicitis'. Under such circumstances there is little justification for mounting an immediate and exhaustive search for the precise underlying cause. All these factors require the ability to tolerate a higher degree of uncertainty than medical students are usually called upon to bear.

The second reason is to be found in the results of a fascinating study by Gale and Marsden (1983), who found – not surprisingly – that registrars were better at making appropriate diagnoses than senior house officers, who in turn were better than medical students. However, they also discovered that all three groups possessed, and were able to apply, the same range of complex diagnostic thinking processes, although their use of particular components did vary. The differences in the groups' respective ability to make diagnoses were due not merely to their levels of knowledge, but mostly to their ability to access (and therefore apply) the knowledge they did possess. They concluded that medical students in general are likely to face difficulties in clinical problem-solving because of their limited ability to perceive and interpret diagnostic problems, irrespective of the clinical context, since the way in which their knowledge is structured in memory is not geared to clinical practice.

The following example, taken from my own teaching experience, highlights the problem: in a clinical problem-solving exercise, a group of ten students was presented with a 55-year-old man who complained of tiredness of 3 months' duration. He was known to have rheumatoid arthritis affecting the small joints. Despite generating an exhaustive and non-discriminatory list of differential diagnoses, ranging from depression to impending myocardial infarction, no member of the group was able to extrapolate from the information given the actual cause of the symptom of tiredness. (He had, in fact, been self-medicating with aspirin for several months.) When asked directly what the side-effects of salicylates were, all the students knew that they could produce occult blood loss from the gastrointestinal tract which could eventually result in iron-deficiency anaemia of sufficient severity to produce tiredness. All the students also knew that salicylates were one of the commonest treatments for rheumatoid arthritis. Their knowledge was locked away in inaccessible compartments, however, since none of them could make the link without prompting. In the teaching situation, prompting is possible; patients, however, are usually not so obliging!

Some common errors

In attempting to generate diagnostic hypotheses, students are prone to exhibit a number of well-recognized errors (Joorabchi, 1989) as follows:

- *Unwarranted fixation on a hypothesis.* This is one of the commonest errors, and 'is characterized by focusing on a particular hypothesis, twisting all data in an attempt to fit it, ignoring competing hypotheses or data that seemed to deny or rule out the diagnosis at hand' (Joorabchi, 1989). It is most important for students to evaluate in a critical and detached manner the extent to which the information they have gathered supports or refutes any diagnostic hypothesis they have generated.
- *Premature closure of hypothesis generation.* This occurs when, prior to considering a number of appropriate diagnostic hypotheses, the student settles on one possibility and 'ceases to search any further, missing other perhaps more important facets of the whole' (Joorabchi, 1989). To avoid making this mistake the reader should try to include all *appropriate* diagnostic hypotheses, bearing in mind the factors of probability, seriousness and treatability.
- *Rule-out syndrome.* This is the converse of the above; the problem here is that the student erects a multiplicity of diagnostic hypotheses. This is usually a consequence of poorly focused history taking. This trait is exhibited by students (and doctors) who possess 'a form of clinical reasoning that places high value on "not missing" or "ruling out" disorders of low probability' (White, 1988). In order to pursue all the identified diagnostic hypotheses, these students and doctors have to perform unfocused physical examinations and an inordinate number of unnecessary laboratory tests as they 'resort to increasingly expensive hospital-based technological interventions [which are] helping to push our health care establishment ever closer to bankruptcy' (White, 1988). To try to overcome this tendency, diagnostic hypotheses in the 'most likely' category should be limited in the first instance to a maximum of five, and in the 'less likely but important to consider' category to a maximum of two. Only if no support is forthcoming for any of these should additional diagnostic hypotheses be generated.

Other errors include:

- Generation of very unlikely hypotheses (e.g. 'novelties')
- Undue retention of initially appropriate hypotheses which are clearly not sustainable in the light of subsequent information obtained
- Promotion of unsupportable hypotheses.

To try to avoid these errors readers should, before including or retaining any diagnostic hypothesis, try to adopt the habit of asking themselves: Does this particular hypothesis seem credible in the given circumstances? (See also Chapter 11.)

Some practical tips to assist in generating diagnoses

- Make use of the stage of 'prediagnostic interpretation' (PDI) (Gale and Marsden, 1983). This can help to direct and narrow the focus of your field of search for likely diagnoses. For example, if a previously well 65-year-old man presented with dyspnoea of sudden onset of 3 hours' duration and is obviously ill, the PDI would indicate that this is an acute condition, likely to be serious and involving the cardio-vascular and/or respiratory systems. This provides you with a convenient starting point for further enquiry and rules out chronic, trivial conditions affecting most other body systems.
- Whether the PDI is helpful or not, it is a sound policy to concentrate your early problem-solving either by *clarifying* the *presenting symptom* (selected by the patient) or the so-called *pivotal symptom* (selected by the doctor). For example, if the presenting/pivotal symptom is pain, certain cardinal features must be elicited (site, character, severity, radiation, precipitating or relieving factors, duration, onset, previous history) and any associated features (for example, breathlessness, sweating, nausea, vomiting, etc.). The answers to such questions will almost invariably lead you to consider more relevant diagnostic hypotheses.
- If you are having difficulty with the spontaneous generation of diagnostic possibilities, the use of *checklists* can often act as a trigger to the memory. Checklists can facilitate the generation of diagnostic possibilities that would otherwise not have been included. The most useful of these checklists are the so-called 'surgical sieve' and the systems and anatomical approaches respectively (Table 3.1). Checklists

Table 3.1 Checklists to aid generation of likely diagnoses

Surgical sieve	Systems approach	Anatomical approach (e.g. to chest pain)
Congenital	Cardiovascular	Skin
Acquired:	Respiratory	Muscle
Traumatic	Gastrointestinal	Bones
Infective	Genitourinary	Pleura
Inflammatory	Musculoskeletal	Lungs
Metabolic	Neurological	Heart
Haematological	Haemopoietic	Oesophagus/stomach
Degenerative		
Psychological		
Iatrogenic		

are also of use when patients present with such vague symptoms that a large and varied number of diagnostic possibilities could account for them. They can provide you with a systematic approach that enables you to narrow the search area and then proceed to make some PDIs or suggest some finite diagnostic possibilities from this field. Whether, and the extent to which, you make use of one or more checklist(s) will be determined by the particular clinical circumstances. For example, the anatomical approach is best suited to a consideration of presentations concerned with pain, whereas the others are best used to tackle vague symptom presentations.

- Finally, in considering diagnostic hypotheses bear in mind the following general guidelines (Joorabchi, 1989):
  - Uncommon manifestations of common conditions are more common than common manifestations of uncommon conditions
  - Simple conditions are caused by simple problems
  - Diverse symptoms and signs are commonly caused by a single disease or entity
- If all else fails, refer to books or journals, or consult colleagues.

The triple diagnosis

In generating diagnostic hypotheses, it is essential to think in physical *and* social *and* psychological terms – the *triple diagnosis*. This is not to suggest that all diseases have physical, social and psychological components in equal measure, nor that all physical diseases have social and psychological causes as well as physical ones. It is simply to provide a reminder that 'the three aspects of the diagnosis should always be considered at each consultation' (Marinker, 1981) – *as appropriate*. For example, it is not sufficient merely to diagnose correctly acne vulgaris in a teenage girl and then restrict treatment to countering the dermatological manifestations of the disease. In these circumstances, it is also essential to consider the impact of the disease both on the patient's psychological development and on her social functioning. Through an awareness of the person who has the disease, you will be reminded of the need to evaluate the extent to which her self-image and self-confidence have been affected, and how this might have brought about social withdrawal at a very important and vulnerable stage of the patient's life. Consequently, a counselling approach may be required in addition to necessary drug therapy.

Use of time as an aid to diagnosis

On occasions, all clinicians adopt a 'wait-and-see' approach as a deliberate diagnostic strategy. The rationale for use of time is to separate out, in the most economic manner, those patients with a high probability of disease from those with a low probability. Most of you will be familiar with the way in which surgeons will postpone overnight the decision as to whether to operate on a patient with suspected appendicitis in the hope that the clinical picture will become clearer. The use of time as a diagnostic tool is particularly suited to general practice because of the high frequency with which spontaneous remissions occur in the many instances when no firm diagnoses can be made. One study confirmed the efficacy of such a policy when 72% of patients who had originally been undiagnosed did not need to return to their doctors, mainly because of spontaneous remission of symptoms (Thomas, 1974). To use time appropriately and effectively, however, doctors must be able to control in themselves − and allay in their patients − the almost inevitable feelings of uncertainty which can arise in the interim.

A general practitioner faced with a patient presenting a problem has to answer the following question: Has this patient got a disease? The three possible answers are 'no', 'yes' and 'not sure'. If the answer is 'no', the doctor will need to determine why the patient has come − is it fear of having developed a certain condition, for example cancer, or does this presentation mask some other underlying problem?

If the doctor believes the patient has a disease but cannot diagnose it, or if the doctor is not sure if the patient has a disease or not, there is the particular opportunity to use time as a diagnostic tool. Whether, and the extent to which, this is possible must be dictated by the particular clinical circumstances. If the patient is not ill, the doctor may use time to discover whether the condition is self-limiting by arranging to review the patient's progress in a few days or weeks. On the other hand, if the patient is ill, it is more likely that the doctor will need to investigate, or arrange referral or admission to hospital, as a matter of some urgency. For example, it may not be appropriate to wait and see when dealing with a drowsy, febrile irritable infant. Although, on the basis of probabilities, an upper respiratory tract infection is a much more likely diagnosis than meningitis, it may not be possible to exclude the latter with confidence on clinical grounds alone. Waiting to see if the child deteriorates or improves would be highly risky − urgent admission to hospital for lumbar puncture should be considered in order to establish the diagnosis.

When practitioners decide to use time as a diagnostic aid, they can employ a further safety net by outlining the likely course of patients' illnesses and advising them to return if there is significant deviation from this prediction, deterioration in their condition or if new symptoms develop. For example, a general practitioner may quite reasonably make a provisional diagnosis of acute gastroenteritis in a young man who presents with a 2-day history of diarrhoea and vomiting accompanied by vague lower abdominal pains. Once satisfied that the patient has an adequate state of hydration and no signs of acute appendicitis, the doctor can advise the patient on appropriate fluid intake for the next 2–3 days. However, by also advising the patient to consult again if the symptoms do not settle, or if the pain becomes worse, the doctor is allowing for the possibility that the patient might be in the early stages of acute appendicitis.

By using time as a deliberate diagnostic strategy in appropriate circumstances, the general practitioner can avoid the following problems:

- Devoting too much time to minor or self-limiting conditions
- Unnecessarily subjecting his patients to inconvenient, painful or costly investigations
- Increasing his patient's anxiety by over-solicitousness
- Referring to hospital too frequently or with an inappropriate degree of urgency.

By such discriminating use of time, a doctor can safely steer a course between the over-reaction of excessive or inappropriate referrals and the under-reaction of ignoring or failing to identify remediable conditions.

Two practical examples of problem-solving

Case 1

A 61-year-old widow presents with a history of 'wetting herself' for the previous 5 days because she 'can't get to the toilet on time'. She had felt 'perfectly well' prior to the onset of her present symptomatology. Her medical records reveal she has no history of significant illness and that she is an infrequent attender.

Initial interpretation
At this stage, the diagnostic possibilities are:
1. *Most likely*
   a. Urinary tract infection
2. *Less likely but important to consider*
   a. Cystocele
   b. Diabetes.

For the following reasons:

1. Sudden onset
2. Short duration of symptoms
3. Elderly female patient
4. Previously well.

Either of the latter two diagnoses *could* present in this way with incontinence in a female patient of this age.

Initial action
Further information needs to be sought by the doctor through selective questioning to attempt to discriminate between the diagnostic possibilities. It transpires that the patient has frequency of micturition at hourly intervals with some dysuria but no nocturia, haematuria, backache or fever. She feels well otherwise. There is no urine loss on coughing, and no family history or other stigmata of diabetes.

Further interpretation
This provides more support for a lower urinary tract infection, despite the absence of nocturia. Cystocele is virtually ruled out, and diabetes becomes even less likely but still cannot be discounted absolutely.

Further action
- No physical examination carried out since likely yield is negligible
- Midstream urine (MSU) sent to laboratory to seek to confirm diagnosis
- Check for glycosuria carried out at the consultation and found to be absent: this virtually ruled out diabetes
- Antibiotic treatment instituted because of:
  the high probability that the underlying cause is a urinary infection
  the distressing nature of symptoms, which the patient would find difficult to tolerate until MSU result became available
- Explanation to the patient, who is asked to attend in 1 week's time so that the situation could be reassessed.

The MSU result revealed significant *Escherichia coli* infection, confirming diagnosis. The patient's symptoms resolved, and a follow-up MSU revealed sterile urine.

If, however, the patient's symptoms had *not* resolved and the MSU result had been negative, the doctor would have had to reconsider the diagnostic possibilities. These would need to include:

- Unusual presentation of cystocele: this would now entail a gynaecological examination when previously it was not justified
- Psychological causes: this would entail a sensitive search for further information about the patient's social and psychological circumstances. Being an infrequent attender, she may be a stoic and therefore reluctant to confess easily to emotional illness. Is her symptomatology connected with her widowhood/family/recent life events?

If none of these diagnostic possibilities was confirmed and the symptoms persisted, the patient would require referral in the first instance to a genitourinary surgeon because the general practitioner has now reached the limits of his competence.

Case 2

The second example illustrates how slight variations in the presenting symptomatology can significantly influence the nature of diagnostic probabilities and the ease with which they can be identified. It also illustrates the variable impact of demographic and social characteristics on the generation and ranking of diagnostic probabilities.

A 32-year-old divorcee with three children presents with one of the following symptom patterns. In each instance she gives a history of having been 'well' until 2 months previously.

- Presentation I
  Irritability
  Tiredness
  Weight loss
  Dislike of hot weather
  Increased sweating
  Palpitations
  Trembling hands
  Increased appetite
- *Presentation II*
  Irritability
  Tiredness
  Increased sweating
  Weight loss
  Palpitations
  Diminished appetite
- *Presentation III*
  Tiredness
  ? weight loss
  Normal appetite.

Presentation I

In presentation I, the single most likely diagnosis is easily recognizable as thyrotoxicosis because most of the classic symptoms of that disease have been elicited. Because of the patient's social circumstances, some doctors might also consider the possibility of co-existing anxiety/depression, but there are no indications to consider other possibilities at this stage. Nevertheless, physical examination is mandatory and should be directed towards attempting to elicit the physical signs of thyrotoxicosis. With such a presentation many of these are likely to be found but, whatever the physical findings, tests of thyroid function must be carried out to seek to confirm the diagnosis.

In due course, laboratory tests confirmed the present of acute thyrotoxicosis. Following appropriate treatment, all symptoms disappeared, indicating that they had a purely physical basis and were not related to the patient's social circumstances.

Presentation II
In presentation II, the diagnostic possibilities are as follows:

1. *Most likely*
   a. Anxiety/depression
   b. Anaemia
   c. Thyrotoxicosis
2. *Less likely but important to consider*
   a. Carcinoma of breast/cervix
   b. Pulmonary tuberculosis.

Thyrotoxicosis has been relegated because the symptoms of dislike of hot weather and shakiness are absent, and weight loss is not accompanied by a good appetite. It still remains a possible diagnosis, however. Anxiety (with or without depression) and anaemia become prime possibilities, because these conditions are relatively common in female patients in this age group and also because of the potential relationship of the symptomatology with the patient's social circumstances.

The search for further information should concentrate on the elicitation of features of depression: for example, feeling low, weepy spells, disturbed sleep pattern, suicidal tendency. Possible reasons for anxiety/depression should also be sought: for example, is the patient in financial difficulty? Are there problems with the children? Is there a new relationship or the ending of an old one? Has she trouble with her ex-husband? With regard to anaemia, enquiry should concentrate on aspects of diet because the patient may be neglecting herself, given her social circumstances. Since she was well until 2 months previously, meno/metrorrhagia is unlikely but should be enquired about, as should information on the colour of the stools. Enquiries should also be made about the presence of night sweats, haemoptysis, blood-stained vaginal discharge and postcoital bleeding with or without dyspareunia.

On physical examination, the general demeanour of the patient should be noted, since in depression affect will be flattened, e.g. her head may be bowed. Physical agitation would support the diagnosis both of anxiety and thyrotoxicosis. The features of anaemia (pallor of mucous membranes, koilonychia) and signs of thyrotoxicosis (tachycardia, sweaty palms, enlarged thyroid gland with bruit, exophthalmos, etc.), should be sought. Examination of the chest, breast and cervix may be required, depending on the particular history obtained. Depending on the physical findings, it may be necessary to carry out haemoglobin and full blood count as well as thyroid function tests.

In the event, all of these were normal, as the patient's problems were due to anxiety/depression precipitated by financial difficulties and behaviour problems with the children. In these circumstances, management may include the use of anxiolytics and antidepressants, a counselling approach from the doctor and a possible contribution from the social worker.

Presentation III
In presentation III, the presenting symptoms are so vague that the number of diagnostic probabilities is very large and likely to vary from no disease present at all to serious underlying pathology. If no further useful information can be elicited from the history, it will be necessary to make some PDIs to try to provide some indication of the degree of urgency involved and the extent to which a further search for possible underlying causes needs to be mounted. For example, if the patient feels or looks ill and objective evidence of weight loss can be elicited, an inductive approach to history, examination and investigations may need to be used. If this proves inconclusive, early referral to hospital is indicated.

Key points

- The primary task of the consultation is to discover what is wrong with the patient.
- Making a diagnosis is a complex process that involves a large number of component skills.
- It is important to understand how diagnoses are reached so that successes may be repeated and failures corrected.
- Although the inductive method is a useful learning framework, the hypothetico-deductive approach to formulating diagnoses is more often used and is more effective in clinical practice.
- The primacy of the history in both the diagnostic process and patient management cannot be over-stressed.
- Diagnostic probabilities are dependent on the clinical context as well as the nature and duration of symptoms and the types of people who experience them.
- Diagnoses should be formulated in physical, psychological and social terms *as appropriate*.
- Although diagnosis often precedes and predicts management, the diagnostic process often includes management, particularly in the setting of general practice.
- Remember: 'It is the quality of thinking and not the quantity of facts that is likely to lead to the resolution of clinical problems' (Marinker, 1976).
- Finally: 'The teacher and the student should pay as much attention to economy as they customarily devote to thoroughness. There need be no conflict between the two' (Campbell, 1987).

References

Barrows, H. S., Norman, G. R., Neufeld V. R. and Feightner J. W. (1982). The clinical reasoning process of randomly selected physicians in general medical practice. *Clinical and Investigative Medicine*, 5, 49.
Campbell, E. J. M. (1987). The diagnosing mind. *Lancet*, April 11 849–51.

Dixon, A. S. (1986). 'There's a lot of it about': clinical strategies in family practice. *Journal of the Royal College of General Practitioners*, **36**, 468–71.

Elstein, A. S., Loupe, M. I. and Erdmonn, J. B. (1971). An experimental study of diagnostic thinking. *Journal of Structural Learning*, **2**, 45.

Elstein. A. S., Shulman. L. S. and Sprafka S. I. (1978). *Medical Problem Solving – An Analysis of Clinical Reasoning*. Cambridge, Massachusetts: Harvard University Press.

Elwyn, G. J. (1997). So many precious stories: a reflective narrative of patient-based medicine in general practice, Christmas 1996. *British Medical Journal*, **315**, 1659.

Federman, D. D. (1990). The education of medical students: sounds, alarums and excursions. *Academic Medicine*, **65**(4), 221–6.

Fraser, R. C. (1994). *The Leicester Assessment Package*, 2nd edn. Glaxo Medical Fellowship.

Gale, J. and Marsden P. (1983). *Medical Diagnosis: From Student to Clinician*. Oxford: Oxford University Press.

Gale, J. and Marsden, P. (1985). Diagnosis: process not product. In *Decision Making in General Practice* (M. Sheldon *et al.*, eds.), Chapter 7. Basingstoke: Macmillan.

Hampton, J. R., Harrison, M. J. B. and Mitchell J. R. A. (1975). Relative contributions of history taking, physical examination and laboratory investigation to diagnosis and management of medical outpatients. *British Medical Journal*, **2**, 486–9.

Hoffbrand, B. I. (1989). Away with the system review: a plea for parsimony. *British Medical Journal*, **298**, 817–19.

Joorabchi, B. (1989). Medical information processing skills: guide posts to clinical assessment. *Medical Teacher*, **11**, 331.

Marinker, M. (1976). Clinical problem-solving in general practice. In *Practice – A Handbook of Primary Medical Care* (J. Cormack, M. Marinker and D. Morrell, eds.). London: Kluwer Medical.

Marinker, M. (1981). Whole person medicine. In *Teaching General Practice* (J. Cormack, M. Marinker and D. Morrell, eds.). London: Kluwer Medical.

Royal College of General Practitioners (1972). *The Future General Practitioner: Learning and Teaching*. London: British Medical Association.

Sandler, G. (1979). Costs of unnecessary tests. *British Medical Journal*, **2**, 21–4.

Sandler, G. (1984). In *Common Medical Problems*, p. 578. Lancaster: MTP Press Limited.

Slovic, P., Fischoff, B. and Lichtenstein, S. (1982). Facts versus fears: understanding perceived risks. In *Judgement under Certainty: Heuristics and Biases* (D. Khaneman, P. Slovic and A. Tuersky, eds.). Cambridge: Cambridge University Press.

Thomas, K. B. (1974). Temporarily dependent patients in general practice. *British Medical Journal*, **1**, 625–6.

van der Vleuten, C. P. M. (1996). The assessment of professional competence: developments, research and practical implications. In *Advances in Health Sciences Education, 1*. The Netherlands: Kluwer Academic Publisher.

White, K. L. (1988). *The Task of Medicine*, p. 45. Menlo Park, California: The Henry J. Kaiser Family Foundation.

4
Patient management
Brian R. McAvoy

Each patient carries his own witch-doctor
inside him. We are at our best when we give
the doctor who resides within each patient a
chance to go to work (Albert Schweizer).

The inter-relationship of diagnosis and management has already been
described in the previous chapter. If diagnosis is the science of clinical
method, then management is the art. The variety and complexity of
problems presented to the general practitioner by the individual patients,
families and practice population he is responsible for allows a wide range
of management options and roles for the doctor. These have been aptly
described by Balint (1986a):

> Should he be a kind of authoritative guardian who knows best what is
> good for his wards, who need give no explanation, but expects loyal
> obedience? Should he act as mentor, offering his expert knowledge and
> ready to teach his patient how to adjust himself to changed conditions,
> how to adopt a new, more useful attitude? Should he be a detached
> scientist, describing objectively the advantages and drawbacks of the
> various therapeutic and dietetic possibilities and allowing his patient
> complete freedom of choice, but also imposing upon him the responsi-
> bility for the choice? Should he act the kind protective parent who must
> spare his poor child-patient any bad tidings or painful responsibility?
> Or should he be an advocate of 'truth above all', firmly believing that
> nothing can be worse than doubt, and acting accordingly? The answer,
> of course, is that the doctor must judge what is best for each patient.

Although management must be geared to the particular problems and
circumstances of individual patients, it is possible, nevertheless, to consider management under the following broad headings:

1. Reassurance and/or explanation
2. Advice
3. Prescription
4. Referral
5. Investigation

6. Observation (follow-up)
7. Prevention.

It must be stressed, however, that these headings are intended simply as an *aide-memoire*. The order in which they are listed does not imply their relative importance and, in some cases, many of the subdivisions may be neither needed nor appropriate. A convenient acronym is RAPRIOP.

The management behaviour of doctors has come under increasing scrutiny over recent years as a result of limited resources, increasing patient demand and burgeoning biotechnology. The general practitioner's role as 'gatekeeper' between primary and secondary care is therefore critical. Management decisions concerning patients have obvious direct effects on those individuals, but also have indirect implications for other patients in the practice and the community at large in terms of resource utilization. Although, like any clinician, the general practitioner's primary responsibility is to the individual patients or families he cares for, he must increasingly be aware of these broader implications of his decision making. Greater public accountability has brought into sharper focus the appropriateness of all aspects of a clinician's activities, and this is likely to be an area of growing importance in the future. Indeed, the White Paper, The New NHS (Department of Health, 1997a), increases responsibilities of British general practitioners for the development of primary and community health care and the shaping of hospital services. Moreover, the development of evidence-based medicine – 'the conscientious, explicit and judicious use of current best evidence in making decisions about the care of individual patients' (Sackett *et al.*, 1997) – has encapsulated and articulated the essence of good clinical practice.

Reassurance and/or explanation

The need for reassurance may be the main reason for the patient presenting to the doctor, and management may and often does consist solely of this. Indeed, as Michael Balint (1986b) said:

> In spite of our almost pathetic lack of knowledge about the dynamisms and possible consequences of 'reassurance' and 'advice', these two are perhaps the most often used forms of medical treatment. In other words they are the most frequent forms in which the drug 'doctor' is administered. What, after all, can be more natural than to sympathize with a patient in distress . . . the patient is often relieved by our sincere 'reassurance' and afterwards, things develop in a favourable direction.

Inappropriate reassurance, however, can be a positive danger to the patient and can damage the doctor–patient relationship along with the doctor's credibility. In the words of Kessel (1979), 'The utterance of reassurance should be as planned and deliberate as the use of any other medical skill'. Furthermore, reassurance also needs to be accompanied by an appropriate degree of explanation.

To many individuals, certain symptoms or signs are strongly suggestive of a specific disease, e.g. chest pains and palpitations – coronary artery disease; backache – slipped disc; headaches and dizziness – high blood pressure or an impending stroke; 'lumps' – cancer. Unless the doctor explores the patients' understanding of their symptoms and their possible significance, it will not be possible to reassure them adequately. For example, Mrs Green, a 46-year-old woman who is a relatively frequent attender with stress-related symptoms, presents with a history of headaches of 3 weeks' duration. Attempting to reassure her that history and examination reveal no abnormality, or telling her that her blood pressure is perfectly normal, will not be successful on this occasion. This is because, unknown to and undiscovered by the doctor, a close friend of Mrs Green had died from a brain tumour a few weeks earlier, having initially presented to her doctor with headaches. If Mrs Green's doctor had been able to ascertain this, it would have been possible to provide specific and therefore effective reassurance. Indeed, with this type of patient, blanket reassurance may exacerbate her anxieties by fuelling her suspicions that she does have a brain tumour and the belief that the doctor is trying to be kind by hiding the true diagnosis from her. In short, doctors must firstly satisfy themselves that they have not only discovered the true nature of a patient's problems, but also that they can safely be managed by reassurance.

Communication and trust are two other factors that influence the success of reassurance as a management technique. First, explaining the problem in terms that the patient can understand is critical. Besides obvious factors such as intelligence and education, the doctor must also take into account medical experience, ethnic background, social class and personality. An articulate, pedantic university lecturer and an illiterate diffident labourer who both suffer symptoms of a hiatus hernia will require explanations which are likely to differ significantly in language, emphasis and detail (see Chapter 6 for further details).

The second influential factor is the degree of trust that the patient has in the doctor. Reassurance carries more weight if there is a strong bond between the doctor and the patient. Continuity of care as provided by the British general practitioner has several advantages, not least of which is the opportunity it provides to nurture and develop a relationship of mutual trust and respect between doctor and patient. A quarter of consultations in general practice involve chronic, incurable conditions such as arthritis, chronic bronchitis and multiple sclerosis. The natural history of these diseases makes repeated consultations inevitable, allowing the doctor–patient relationship to develop. This so-called 'mutual investment company' (Balint, 1986c) is of particular significance in these conditions where care takes precedence over cure (see Chapter 5).

Case history

Barbara Marston, aged 58 years, had a major right-sided stroke 2 years ago. She was hospitalized for 3 months, and remains considerably disabled with dysphasia and a hemiparesis. She can walk short distances with a caliper and tripod, and has good support from her husband. Six months previously she had to be readmitted to hospital with a deep vein thrombosis in her right calf, an event she resented, since she interpreted it as a 'set back' in her rehabilitation. She insists on attending the surgery for her 3-monthly checks and always sees the doctor who originally admitted her to hospital. She attends today, 6 weeks before her regular check is due, complaining of discomfort in her left calf. The doctor diagnoses a superficial thrombophlebitis and advises analgesia and an elastic support, reassuring her that there is no evidence of a deep vein thrombosis and no need for her to be readmitted. His reassurance and explanation are accepted with trust and relief.

The doctor can be confident in his diagnosis and management because he has examined Mrs Marston's legs on several occasions and knows her fear of having to be rehospitalized. The patient's past experiences and continuing relationship with the doctor have enhanced her trust in him, and makes it easier for her to accept his judgement. Moreover, this further episode increases the stocks of both the doctor and the patient in the 'mutual investment company'.

As previously mentioned in Chapter 2, evidence is accumulating that such interpersonal aspects of the consultation can influence not only patient satisfaction and compliance but also health outcomes (Kaplan *et al.*, 1989), This is considered further in Chapters 5, 6 and 8.

Advice

Here, the concepts of whole-person medicine and continuity of care are essential to effective management. As with diagnoses, management should be considered in terms of physical, emotional and social aspects, where appropriate. Continuity of care enables problems to be seen in perspective, and often makes the general practitioner the most appropriate health professional to advise individuals on their lifestyle and behaviour (McCron and Budd, 1979).

To be effective, advice must be realistically geared to the patient's circumstances and lifestyle. For example, a flexible shift worker would find it easier to take a single bedtime dose of an antidepressant rather than three smaller doses spread throughout the working day. Standard and 'routine' advice may have to be modified considerably for the individual patient. The general practitioner is in a unique position to tailor his management to the personality and circumstances of the individual.

Case history

Derick Hardwick is a 55-year-old former headmaster of a school for the mentally handicapped. Following a turbulent marriage and divorce, he remarried 3 years ago and began renovating a barge to use in his retirement. Previously well, he has within the last twelve months sustained two myocardial infarctions, forcing his early retirement and leaving him with moderately severe angina despite the use of calcium antagonists, long-acting nitrates, betablockers and aspirin. Coronary arteriography has revealed generalized atheromatous disease, but no specific lesions amenable to angioplasty or bypass surgery. He feels angry, cheated and frustrated at his physical limitations. Conventional medicine now has nothing left to offer him. However, his confidence and morale are improving because his doctor has encouraged him to devote his energies to finishing the barge, advice that on the face of it might seem detrimental to his health. For Derick Hardwick, the conventional advice to 'slow down and take things easy' would have been totally inappropriate, undermining further his battered confidence.

Counselling

Sometimes reassurance, advice and explanation are insufficient, and the doctor may be required to assume a more formal counselling role to help patients work through or come to terms with their problems. Counselling has been defined as 'the various techniques and methods by which people can be helped to understand themselves and to be more effective' (Munro *et al.*, 1988). A more comprehensive definition is 'the skilled and principled use of relationships which develop self-knowledge, emotional acceptance and growth, and personal resources. The overall aim is to live more fully and satisfyingly. Counselling may be concerned with addressing and resolving specific problems, making decisions, coping with crises, working through feelings and inner conflict, or improving relationships with others. The counsellor's role is to facilitate the client's work in ways that respect the client's values, personal resources, and capacity for self-determination' (BAC, 1992).

The fundamental aim of counselling is to assist patients to identify and implement their own unique solutions to a particular problem. This is done by helping patients not only to develop insight into their particular situation, but also to identify the range of possible courses of action open to them from which they can make a choice. Implicit in counselling is the recognition by patients that they will be required to modify their behaviour. Counselling is therefore more than just giving advice, but falls short of psychotherapy. Nevertheless, effective counselling provides comfort to the patient and can result in demonstrable improvements in physical and mental well-being and health.

Different levels of involvement in the counselling role will be required, depending on the nature of the problem(s) presented or uncovered. Some patients will realize that they are not physically or mentally ill, but recognize that they are having difficulty in adapting to, or coping with problems in their day-to-day life: for example, an unhappy woman whose husband is having an affair, the confused parents of rebellious teenage children or the lonely mother who cannot reconcile herself to the marriage and subsequent emigration to Australia of her only daughter. These patients are aware of the underlying cause of their distress and are seeking mainly comfort and support.

Alternatively, patients may present with physical symptoms, the underlying cause of which may be related to work or relationship problems. The patients, however, lack the insight to be able to make the appropriate connection: for example, the over-stressed business man whose symptoms are tiredness and dyspepsia, or the obsessive teacher who develops palpitations and insomnia on promotion to a position of higher responsibility. In these instances, the doctor will need first of all to help the patient to develop the necessary insight as a prelude to seeking solutions. In these situations, counselling can play a vital role in the prevention of somatic fixation.

The extent to which counselling is undertaken personally by an individual doctor varies greatly, and is dependent on both the doctor's level of inclination and skill. Many doctors, while recognizing the need for counselling, prefer to refer patients in need to non-medical personnel such as community psychiatric nurses or psychologists. Over the past decade many counsellors have become members of primary health care teams and work within the practice premises.

Prescription

Prior to outlining the factors that must be considered before a doctor issues a prescription, it should be remembered that twice as many medicines are taken by patients on their own initiative (so-called 'over-the-counter' medicines) as are prescribed by a doctor (Wright and MacAdam, 1979; see also Chapter 1). One study found that 80% of a random sample of adults interviewed had taken some form of medicine in the previous 2 weeks, although only 16% of this group had consulted a doctor (Dunnell and Cartwright, 1972). To minimize the occurrence of unwanted interactions between prescribed and self-administered drugs it is therefore wise to check if a patient has been taking self-medication and, if so, what drug, for how long and with what effect.

As with other aspects of management, such as referral and investigation, prescribing must take into account patients' expectations and their autonomy, and this often involves negotiation with the patient. For example, a young man who comes complaining of 'feeling all tensed up' may expect or even request 'something to calm me down', but after appropriate explanation and reassurance may well be happy to accept advice on relaxation exercises. Whether or not a prescription is issued, it should always be made clear to patients that they are free to return if they are not satisfied with the advice offered.

The cost of prescriptions in the National Health Service in England in 1996–97 was £4.5 billion, i.e. about 11% of NHS expenditure (Prescription Pricing Authority, 1997). General practitioners account for over three-quarters of all NHS prescribing costs and, in 1996, 58% of prescriptions were written generically. The number of NHS items dispensed each year has increased steadily, while the proportion of prescriptions exempt from charge increased from 76% to 86% between 1986 and 1996. In England, between 1987 and 1996, the number of prescription items dispensed per person per year rose from just over seven to 9.9 (Department of Health, 1997b). In 1996, the most frequently prescribed drugs were for the cardiovascular system (19%), the nervous system (18%), infections (10%) and respiratory disorders (10%). On average, general practitioners issue prescriptions in two-thirds of their face-to-face consultations (Fraser and Gosling, 1985), but the range is considerable (40–97%). A study of computerized prescribing in seven practices in England (Purves and Kennedy 1994) found that 65% of all prescriptions were 'repeats', i.e. issued without a consultation (range = 54–72%).

The decision whether to prescribe or not in a consultation is critical. Before issuing any prescription, there are some simple questions you should ask yourself (based on Wright and MacAdam, 1979):

1. *What are the clinical aims of prescribing for this particular patient?*
   a. Therapeutic?
      i. Preventive, e.g. antibiotic use prior to dental extraction in a patient with known rheumatic heart disease.
      ii. Curative, e.g. malathion lotion for scabies.
      iii. Symptomatic, e.g. non-steroidal anti-inflammatory agent for osteoarthrosis.
   b. Tactical?
      i. To gain time when collecting more information, e.g. an antacid for a patient with dyspepsia who is awaiting endoscopy.
      ii. To maintain contact with the patient, e.g. when asking a patient to return after a specified period of time on a drug to give a progress report – this allows a check on compliance, enables the doctor to assess efficacy and possible side-effects, and can nurture the doctor–patient relationship. An example is an asymptomatic middle-aged man on anti-hypertensive therapy.
      iii. As a trial of treatment – e.g. a course of disodium cromoglycate in a young man with a history suggestive of exercise-induced asthma. If successful, the treatment could be maintained.

iv. To relieve the doctor's anxiety when there may be clinical uncertainty – e.g. a systemic antibiotic plus antihistamine for an acute inflammatory lesion of a limb that could be infective or allergic or both.

c. Both?

Examples b) (i), (iii) and (iv) also have therapeutic aims.

2. *What evidence is there that the natural history of this problem will be helped by any medication?*

Many patients expect the doctor to prescribe antibiotics for upper respiratory tract infections. Systematic reviews and individual studies indicate that the evidence in favour of prescribing antibiotics for most presentations of sore throat in general practice is at best marginal, and the benefits are probably outweighed by the likely cost and side-effects of the antibiotics. (Little and Williamson, 1996). Although it may take longer to explain the reasons for not prescribing than to write a prescription for penicillin, the time and effort invested may be rewarded by producing a modification in that patient's future health-seeking behaviour. The patient may, on developing another sore throat, follow your advice and take soluble aspirin or, indeed, no medication at all. Prescribing an antibiotic in these circumstances merely reinforces the patient's belief in the necessity of such treatment every time such symptoms develop. Similar arguments apply to the prescribing of expectorants for coughs, and of tonics for post-viral debility.

3. *In prescribing any drug or drugs:*

a. What evidence is available regarding:

i. Comparative effectiveness? For example, loop diuretics such as frusemide and bumetanide are more potent than thiazides in patients with cardiac failure. However, for most other groups of drugs, very little information is available on comparative effectiveness. Rational selection can therefore be difficult in certain groups where a choice is extensive, e.g. the current British National Formulary (BNF) lists 23 different non-steroidal anti-inflammatory agents (NSAIDs) and 27 different combined oral contraceptives.

ii. Comparative hazards? It must not be forgotten that drugs are one of the prime factors in iatrogenic disease, a common cause for admissions to hospital, especially amongst the elderly. The BNF and the Data Sheet Compendium provide information on precautions, side-effects and special risk groups. For example, drowsiness is a well-recognized side-effect of antihistamines, but this seems to be less of a problem with the newer preparations such as astemizole and terfenadine (although they can have other side-effects and interactions).

iii. Comparative cost? As a rule, generic preparations cost less than proprietary drugs. The BNF quotes relative price bands for all preparations as a basis for comparison. Sometimes the differences are startling; for example, there is a six-fold difference in price between bendrofluazide B.P. and one of its proprietary forms. Although generic prescribing has other advantages and disadvantages, on balance the case for generic prescribing is stronger than the case against (Consumers' Association, 1987).

b. What are the contraindications to their use?
   As with precautions and side-effects, the BNF and the Data Sheet Compendium provide information on contraindications. One relatively common contraindication, especially to antibiotics, is a previous allergic reaction. Labelling the front of the patient's medical record envelope with a red warning sticker can serve as a useful reminder to the doctor on future occasions when a similar prescription is contemplated.

c. What interactions are to be avoided?
   The risk of interactions increases exponentially with the number of drugs prescribed. It is impossible for a doctor to be aware of all possible interactions, especially with less commonly prescribed preparations. A special appendix in the BNF lists potentially harmful interactions that are likely to have clinical importance. Useful drug interaction card indices, wall charts, discs and 'slide rules' are available from some pharmaceutical companies.

d. What factors influence optimal dosage and duration?
   These include timing relative to meals, body weight, age, route of administration, half-life of the drugs, renal or hepatic impairment and drug interactions.

4. *What factors are likely to affect the patient's compliance?*
   Rates of non-compliance with medication regimes vary from 8–95%, with an average of 40–50% (Ley, 1988). The contributory factors are further discussed in Chapters 5 and 6.

5. *What arrangements, if any, are needed for further supervision?*
   This is of particular relevance with psychotropics (especially hypnotics and anxiolytics), analgesics and skin preparations, which can easily and inappropriately become repeat prescriptions. Two ways of reducing the likelihood of a drug becoming a repeat prescription by default are, first, to decide on the time limit at the initial consultation (and tell the patient this) and, second, to arrange to see the patient again for review.

If in doubt whether or not to give a drug – don't.

The doctor's task is not over once the decision has been made to issue a prescription – there is the obligation to explain a number of matters to the patient:

- Why the prescription has been made
- The importance of taking the drug

- Instructions on taking the drug; when, how often, for how long and by what route
- The expected action and benefits of the drug
- Any likely possible side-effects and what to do if they occur
- Precautions and possible interactions with other drugs, alcohol, etc.
- Instructions on follow-up or renewal of the prescription, if appropriate.

Accurate and reliable sources of information are essential to enable the practitioner to answer many of the questions posed above and to keep abreast of current developments in therapeutics. The *BNF*, the *Drug and Therapeutics Bulletin* (published by the Consumers' Association), *Medicines Resource Centre (MeReC) Bulletins* and the *Prescribers' Journal* are excellent resources. In addition, established journals such as the *Lancet, British Medical Journal, British Journal of General Practice* and the *New England Journal of Medicine* publish regular articles and reviews on drugs. Throughout the country, a network of Drug Information Centres provides expert opinion and advice on any questions or problems related to drugs. Furthermore, regular detailed information on their individual prescribing is now sent quarterly by the Prescription Pricing Authority to all general practitioners in England through the Prescribing Analysis and Cost (PACT) system (Harris *et al.*, 1990). This is intended to promote critical self-appraisal and encourage rational and cost-effective prescribing.

A recent and growing trend has been the compilation of local drug formularies by groups of general practitioners, for example in the UK (Grant *et al.*, 1990) and New Zealand (Toop, 1989). In addition to its educational benefits, this practice should lead to more consistent, rational, safe and economic prescribing (van Zwanenberg, 1986). A recent study showed that, following the development of a formulary for NSAIDs, practices prescribed from a narrower range of drugs and focused a greater proportion of their prescribing on their three most commonly used drugs (Avery *et al.*, 1997).

Referral

Although they deal with the majority of their patients by themselves, general practitioners may refer patients to other individuals or agencies when appropriate. These include:

- General practitioner colleagues or partners with special interests or expertise.
- Other members of the primary health care team – community nurses, health visitors, social workers, counsellors, dieticians, chiropodists.
- Helping agencies, e.g. Age Concern, Relate, Alcoholics Anonymous, Benefits Agency.
- Hospital consultants – as outpatients or inpatients.

The European Study of Referrals from Primary to Secondary Care (COMAC-HSR, 1992) found a UK referral rate of 47.2 per 1000 consultations. Seventy per cent of these were for outpatients, 12% for inpatients, 8% private, 5% through accident and emergency departments and the remainder through clinics or following domiciliary visits by hospital consultants.

Referral rates vary enormously between different practices and different doctors, ranging from less than 1% of all consultations to more than 20% (Wilkin and Smith, 1987). Allowing for random variation and the small numbers in some of the studies, it seems safe to assume that the real variation in GP referral rates is at least three- or four-fold (Roland and Coulter, 1992). These extensive variations in referral rates cannot be explained on the basis of practice size, location, consultation rates, differences in social class or age–sex distribution, or on the age, qualifications or experience of general practitioners, the partnership size or access to diagnostic services. More significant factors may be the general practitioner's temperament (e.g. the ability to tolerate uncertainty), attitude to illness and the value of hospital care, and relationship with hospital colleagues (RCGP and BMA, 1979). You should be aware that you will also be subject to the same influences. There are, however, many problems in measuring general practitioners' rates of referral, and these problems need to be understood before the rates can be interpreted (Roland and Coulter, 1992).

General practitioners refer patients to hospital for a number of reasons, for example:

- To obtain specialist treatment, e.g. surgery or dialysis.
- To obtain a specialist opinion on diagnosis and/or management of a difficult problem. Here the hospital specialist is fulfilling his role as a consultant – e.g. when the general practitioner asks a physician for an opinion on a middle-aged business man with atypical chest pain in order to distinguish between a cardiovascular or gastro-intestinal cause. Such a referral serves to reassure both doctor and patient.
- To gain access to certain diagnostic and therapeutic facilities that may not be available outside hospital, e.g. colonoscopy, echocardi-ography.
- To accede to patients' or relatives' anxiety or pressure – the not un-commonly requested 'second opinion' – e.g. asking a psychiatrist to confirm your diagnosis of depression and advice on further manage-ment for a middle-aged woman with multiple somatic complaints who has only partly responded to antidepressants and whose husband feels that 'something must be done'.
- To provide reinforcement of advice given to a poorly-compliant patient. Sometimes the perceived greater authority of a hospital 'specialist' can have more impact than the general practitioner alone.

Multiple admissions or outpatient attendances can be confusing to patients, especially if they see different doctors on each occasion. This is accentuated by the fact that individuals re-attending outpatient clinics tend to be seen by the more junior hospital doctors, who commonly rotate from post to post at 6-monthly intervals or less. Misunderstandings about diagnosis, prognosis and treatment can easily arise, and these are often compounded by the natural anxieties many individuals experience on attending hospitals. The more individuals involved in the care of the patient, the greater the potential for confusion and conflicting advice. The general practitioner has a crucial role to play here, acting as a reference point, co-ordinator and source of information and explanation. The concepts of whole person medicine and continuity of care are of particular relevance in those patients who have frequent or varied contact with hospital services. For example, a diabetic with osteoarthrosis may be attending a physician, an ophthalmologist, an orthopaedic surgeon and a dietician. The general practitioner's tasks here are to ensure that the varied and extensive expertise available is fully utilized to the patient's benefit, to minimize contradictory advice, to be the patient's advocate and to ensure that the patient understands why these referrals have been made. The general practitioner can also take the longer-term view of the patient and any personal circumstances, balancing physical, social and psychological factors as appropriate and considering both the diagnosis and prognosis – the very essence of continuity of care.

Investigation

Investigations can be performed for a number of reasons, some diagnostic, others therapeutic (House, 1983):

- To confirm or to make more precise a diagnosis suspected from the history and examination, e.g. thyroid function tests in a young woman presenting with weight loss and a goitre.
- To exclude an unlikely but important and treatable disease, e.g. a plasma viscosity in an elderly woman with pains and stiffness in the shoulder girdle muscles, who may have polymyalgia rheumatica.
- To monitor the effects or side-effects of medicine, e.g. haemoglobin and reticulocyte count in a woman with pernicious anaemia commencing on vitamin B12 injections.
- To screen asymptomatic patients, e.g. cervical cytology in sexually active women.
- To reassure an anxious patient that nothing is seriously wrong, e.g. plasma viscosity and rheumatoid factor in a young woman with vague aches and pains, whose mother is crippled with rheumatoid arthritis.
- To convince a sceptical patient that something is wrong and that lifestyle amendments should be made, e.g. liver function tests in a heavy drinker.

The decision to investigate a patient, as with the decision to refer, is based on clinical judgement, which is influenced by many factors – the clinical findings on history and examination (including social and psychological factors), the doctor's temperament and attitudes, the doctor–patient relationship, and organizational factors such as the availability of diagnostic services, the time of day or night, etc. Such decisions are often finely balanced. For example, a 52-year-old man presents with 2 days' coughing accompanied by the production of green sputum streaked with fresh blood. Physical examination is unremarkable. The most likely diagnosis is acute bronchitis, but a less likely and important diagnosis to exclude is bronchial carcinoma. The decision whether or not to order a chest X-ray will depend not only on the doctor's estimate of the relative probabilities (based on smoking history, past history of respiratory problems and response to a course of antibiotics) but also on 'softer' factors, such as the patient's degree of anxiety (one of his relatives or friends may recently have been found to have lung cancer).

As with hospital referrals, doctors vary enormously in their rates of investigation: from 15 to 265 per 1000 consultations, with a mean of 115 (Crombie and Fleming, 1988). General practitioners, however, are very discriminating in their use of laboratory and technical facilities, requesting mainly simple and straightforward tests and achieving a high proportion of abnormal results (Patterson et al., 1974).

If a doctor is still in considerable doubt about the diagnosis after taking a history and examining the patient, it is unlikely that laboratory investigations will be very helpful. Indeed Sandler (1979), in a study of 630 hospital medical outpatients, found that routine blood count, ESR, blood urea and serum electrolyte estimations and urine examinations in the absence of any clinical indication were of minimal value, contributing to only 1% of all diagnoses. He concluded that 'the justification for any investigation should surely be to answer the specific clinical question relating to diagnoses and management only when there is doubt as to either'. A similar study (Sandler, 1984) of emergency tests carried out on 555 patients presenting at hospital with acute medical problems revealed that only 17% of the tests were abnormal and, of these, only one-third helped in treatment and less than one-third helped in diagnosis. Both studies emphasized the considerable cost of indiscriminate investigation, and stressed the over-riding importance of a good clinical history (see Chapter 3). It has been reported that 'a definite and sustained reduction in inappropriate requests for laboratory investigations may be achieved by an ongoing policy of intervention, including issuing guidelines and factsheets and holding seminars, but a positive attitude among senior consultant staff is crucial' (Bareford and Hayling, 1990). In this study a reduction of over 20% in requests for haematological tests was achieved, and this persisted over the ensuing 2 years. Moreover, reducing the volume of GPs' diagnostic tests through feedback does not lead to more specialist referrals (Winkens *et al.*, 1995).

The inappropriateness of 'routine' investigations is probably even greater in general practice since most patients suffer from non-life-threatening, self-limiting conditions.

Scientific method involves critical thought, not uncritical investigation (Fleming and Zilva, 1981). Although it is over 40 years since Richard Asher (1954) listed the questions clinicians should ask themselves before requesting an investigation, they still merit as much consideration today:

- Why am I ordering this test?
- What am I going to look for in the result?
- If I find it, will it affect my diagnosis?
- How will this affect my management of the case?
- Will this ultimately benefit the patient?

In general, investigations should be performed only when the following criteria are satisfied:

- The consequence of the result of the investigation could not be obtained by a cheaper, less intrusive method, e.g. taking a more focused history or using time
- The risks of the investigation should relate to the value of the information likely to be gained
- The result will directly assist in the diagnosis or have an effect on subsequent management.

Observation

Follow-up implies continuing observation at the instigation of the doctor and with the agreement of the patient. It is a part of general practice that is potentially very efficient in that it is possible for the patient to make further appointments easily and as frequently as necessary. However, the onus is usually placed on the patient to remember to come. For many problems, reassurance, explanation and follow-up are the only parts of management which are necessary.

Follow-up is an integral part of the general practitioners' role, embracing all three types of morbidity encountered in their daily work. For minor, self-limiting conditions (52% of consultations), such as gastrointestinal upsets and upper respiratory tract infections, no formal follow-up is required. However, the doctor usually advises the patient to return if there is no improvement within a set period of time or if there is any dramatic change in the condition. This simple strategy eliminates from follow-up those patients with transient illness, but provides a safety net to pick up those patients whose symptoms may presage more serious illness. Acute, major, life-threatening conditions (15% of consultations) such as myocardial infarction and cancers often involve hospitalization, but follow-up on discharge is almost always necessary as a result of the long-term implications of such conditions.

Follow-up is of paramount importance for the chronic incurable problems that constitute 33% of a general practitioner's workload. Here, the diagnosis has already been made and the emphasis is on care, not cure. Regular supervision and periodic reassessment of patients with such conditions as hypertension, diabetes and epilepsy are the cornerstones of good clinical practice: therapy can be reviewed, compliance checked and possible complications anticipated or identified at an early and remediable stage (see Chapter 7). At present, some patients attend hospital outpatient clinics for years, seeing a different junior hospital doctor at each visit. The value of this costly exercise is doubtful, and it is likely that, in time, more of these patients will be cared for entirely by general practitioners, who are better placed to provide continuity of care. Such an approach also encourages the development of a good doctor–patient relationship, with its inherent benefits (see Chapter 5).

Excessive follow-up and over-solicitousness, however, can be counterproductive by reducing patients' responsibility for their health and eroding their independence. A good practitioner will achieve the right balance between responsive and anticipatory care, whilst respecting patients' autonomy.

Prevention

Prevention, care and cure are all part of anticipatory care, which encompasses both health promotion and disease prevention. Preventive advice relating to the presenting problem(s) should always form part of your management plan, e.g. advice on lifting for patients presenting with backache. Furthermore, the setting of general practice and the role of the general practitioner provide unique opportunities for opportunistic anticipatory care, i.e. preventive opportunities not related to the presenting complaint(s) – e.g. offering to check the blood pressure of a middle-aged man attending with a musculoskeletal injury. Such actions can improve the health status of the population by offering an answer to our present killing and disabling diseases (see Chapters 7 and 8).

Key points

Patient management can be considered under the following broad headings:

- Reassurance and/or explanation
  Must be specific and related to the patient's perception of the problem. Its success as a management technique depends on communication and trust.
- Advice
  Must be tailored to the personality and circumstances of the individual patient.
- Prescription
  The decision whether to prescribe or not must take into account patient's expectations and autonomy. The clinical aims of prescribing can be therapeutic, tactical or both. If in doubt whether or not to give a drug – don't.
- Referral
  Whenever a referral is made, the general practitioner should act as a reference point, co-ordinator and source of information and explanation for the patient, drawing together the skills associated with whole person medicine and continuity of care.
- Investigation
  Investigations should be considered in terms of their cost–benefit and risks, and should be performed only when their results will directly assist in the diagnosis or have an effect on subsequent management.
- Observation
  Ensures that a doctor can monitor a patient's clinical progress and take any appropriate action.
- Prevention
  Involves health promotion and disease prevention; these are increasingly important in clinical practice in reducing premature death and disability.

References

Asher, R. (1954). Straight and crooked thinking in medicine. *British Medical Journal*, **2**, 460.

Avery, A. J., Walker, B., Heron, T. and Teasdale, S. (1997). Do prescribing formularies help GPs prescribe from a narrower range of drugs? A controlled trial of the introduction of prescribing formularies for NSAIDs. *British Journal of General Practice*, **47**, 810.

BAC (1992). *Code of Ethics and Practice for Counsellors*. Rugby: British Association for Counselling.

Balint, M. (1986a). *The Doctor, His Patient and The Illness*, p. 228. Edinburgh: Churchill Livingstone.

Balint, M. (1986b). *The Doctor, His Patient and The Illness*, p. 116. Edinburgh: Churchill Livingstone.

Balint, M. (1986c). *The Doctor, His Patient and The Illness*, p. 249. Edinburgh: Churchill Livingstone.

Bareford, D. and Hayling, A. (1990). Inappropriate use of laboratory services: long term combined approach to modify request patterns. *British Medical Journal*, **301**, 1305.

COMAC-HSR (1992). *The European Study of Referrals from Primary to Secondary Care*. London: Royal College of General Practitioners.

Consumers' Association (1987). For and against generic prescribing. *Drug and Therapeutic Bulletin*, **25**, 93.

Crombie, D. L. and Fleming, D. M. (1988). *Practice Activity Analysis*. Occasional Paper 41. London: Royal College of General Practitioners.

Department of Health (1997a). *The New NHS. Modern. Dependable*. London: The Stationery Office.

Department of Health (1997b). *Statistics of Prescriptions Dispensed in the Community: England 1986 to 1996*. London: Department of Health.

Dunnell, K. and Cartwright A. (1972). *Medicine Takers, Prescribers and Hoarders*. London: Routledge and Kegan Paul.

Fleming P. R. and Zilva J. F. (1981). Work-loads in chemical pathology: too many tests? *Health Trends*, **13**, 46.

Fraser, R. C. and Gosling, J. T. L. (1985). Information systems for general practitioners for quality assessment: III. Suggested new prescribing profile. *British Medical Journal*, **291**, 1613.

Grant, G. B., Gregory, D. A. and van Zwanenberg, T. D. (1990). *A Basic Formulary for General Practice*, 2nd edn. Oxford: Oxford University Press.

Harris, C. M., Heywood, P. L. and Clayden, A. D. (1990). *The Analysis of Prescribing in General Practice. A Guide to Audit and Research*. London: HMSO.

House, W. (1983). What's in a test? *Update*, **27**, 372.

Kaplan, S. H., Greenfield, S. and Ware, J. E. (1989). Assessing the effects of patient–physician interactions on the outcomes of chronic disease. *Medical Care*, **27**, S110.

Kessel, N. (1979). Reassurance. *Lancet*, **1**, 1128.

Ley, P. (1988). *Communicating with Patients. Improving Communication, Satisfaction and Compliance*, pp. 70–71. London: Croom Helm.

Little, P. and Williamson, I. (1996). Sore throat management in general practice. *Family Practice*, **13**, 317.

McCron, R. and Budd, J. (1979). Communication and health education – a preliminary study. Unpublished document prepared for the Health Education Council, Chapter 8. University of Leicester Centre for Mass Communication Research.

Munro, E. A., Manthei, R. J. and Small, J. J. (1988). *Counselling: The Skills of Problem Solving*. Auckland: Longman Paul.

Patterson, H. R., Fraser, R. C. and Peacock, E. (1974). Diagnostic procedures and the general practitioner. *Journal of the Royal College of General Practitioners*, **24**, 237.

Prescription Pricing Authority (1997). *Annual Report 1996–1997*. Newcastle upon Tyne: Prescription Pricing Authority.

Purves, I. and Kennedy, J. (1994). *The Quality of General Practice Repeat Prescribing*. Newcastle upon Tyne: Sowerby Unit for Primary Care Informatics.

Roland, M. and Coulter, A. (1992). *Hospital Referrals*. Oxford General Practice Series, no. 23. Oxford: Oxford University Press.

Royal College of General Practitioners and the British Medical Asociation (1979). *Trends in General Practice*, p. 91. London: British Medical Association.

Sackett, D. L., Richardson, W. S., Rosenberg, W. and Haynes, R. B. (1997). *Evidence-based Medicine. How to Practice and Teach EBM*, p. 2. Edinburgh: Churchill Livingstone.

Sandler, G. (1979). Costs of unnecessary tests. *British Medical Journal*, **2**, 21.

Sandler, G. (1984). Do emergency tests help in the management of acute medical admissions? *British Medical Journal*, **289**, 973.

Toop, L. (ed.) (1989). *General Practice Preferred Medicines List*. Christchurch: Canterbury Faculty, Royal New Zealand College of General Practitioners, Department of Community Health and General Practice, Christchurch School of Medicine.

van Zwanenberg, T. D. (1986). Prescribing in general practice. In *The Royal College of General Practitioners Members' Reference Book*, pp. 254–6. London: Royal College of General Practitioners.

Wilkin, D. and Smith, A. (1987). Explaining variations in general practitioner referrals to hospital. *Family Practice*, **4**, 160.

Winkens, R. A. G., Grol, R. P. T .M., Beusmans G. H. M .I. *et al.*, (1995). Does a reduction in general practitioners' use of diagnostic tests lead to more hospital referrals? *British Journal of General Practice*, **45**, 289.

Wright, J. J., MacAdam, D. B. (1979). Clinical thinking and practice: diagnosis and decision in patient care. Edinburgh:Churchill Livingstone, pp 146–153.

5

The doctor–patient relationship

Pauline A. McAvoy

The most extraordinary social contract in
human history, the doctor–patient
relationship (Federman 1990).

In this chapter, the characteristics and consequences of this relationship, both good and bad, will be described. In doing so it is hoped to demonstrate that the doctor–patient relationship is neither a luxury nor an optional extra, but an integral component of clinical method and practice, whether in hospital or general practice.

What's it all about?

The doctor–patient relationship is the subject of an extensive literature which provides insights from psychodynamic, behavioural and sociological perspectives. At best, the doctor–patient relationship should be one of trust, mutual respect and empathy. Empathy means putting oneself imaginatively into someone else's position, and understanding the feelings which doing so arouses. A good relationship takes time to develop and is something more than common courtesy and concern, which are social rather than professional skills. As students, you will frequently observe such a relationship but will rarely experience it, in all its facets, for yourselves.

Brown and Pedder (1979) describe this special relationship as having three elements – *a therapeutic or working alliance, transference and countertransference*.

The *therapeutic alliance* refers to the good working relationship that is necessary for any transaction to be successful. It is characterized by friendliness, courtesy and reliability. In medicine, this would be described as establishing a good rapport with the patient. Achieving this stage of the relationship is well within the capabilities of every student, and you should aim to do so in each consultation in which you participate.

Transference refers to a phenomenon readily ascribed to psychother-apy, but which, in general terms, occurs when we respond to a new relationship according to patterns from the past. There is a tendency in us all to carry over into the present attitudes and impressions gained from similar past experiences; thus the doctor may be seen in the patient's imagination as an over-controlling parent or an idealized son.

Eric Berne (1973) describes our being able to take up one of three stances in our interactions with each other – parent, child and adult. In this model of human behaviour, each one of us is able to occupy these three roles and to switch between one and another according to the situation and the person with whom we are interacting.

An example of this might be the plump, middle-aged lady who says with a coy smile, 'You'll be very angry with me, doctor, I haven't lost a single pound this week. I've been very naughty'. Here, the child is inviting the doctor to behave as a reproving parent. The doctor can, of course, respond by chastizing her, or may choose more effectively to turn the transaction into an adult one and discuss with the patient why she finds such difficulty in controlling her weight.

Anxiety about illness may encourage a patient to regress to childlike levels of functioning and to react to a doctor as a parent or authority figure. This may of course be very appropriate behaviour, for example in acute life-threatening illness, but such behaviour would normally subside once the acute phase resolved. Later on we will look at the implications for the doctor–patient relationship when this behaviour persists.

The third element which Brown and Pedder describe in the doctor–patient relationship is that of *countertransference*. This refers to the feelings that doctors have towards their patients. Most doctors are aware of the profound feeling of depression that can be generated within themselves when talking to a depressed patient, but what of anger, sadness, guilt, compassion and irritation? Sometimes students and doctors feel that it is wrong to have and to show such feelings. They believe, and have often been taught, that they should somehow be able to rise above them. For example, a senior medical student, bored with clerking 'yet another diarrhoea', handed over the next admission to a fellow student while he awaited 'something more interesting'. This turned out to be a 4-year-old child with headaches, who was sub-sequently found to have a malignant cerebral tumour. The student found himself completely unable to discuss the diagnosis with the distressed mother, afraid that he might cry. Later, he described his feelings of inadequacy and his anger at the system which had taught him about the 'interesting' case, but not how to deal with his own emotions or those of patients and their relatives.

The recognition of the feelings engendered in us by our patients may be as important a diagnostic sign as a rapid pulse or finger-clubbing. Browne and Freeling (1976) refer to the emotional experience evoked in the examining doctor by the attitude and bearing of the patient as the 'sixth sense'. It follows, therefore, that doctors should understand their own feelings and be able to modify their expressions – to understand others one must know oneself:

> If awareness of feelings is suppressed, then not only may important information be lost to view, but incorrect action may be taken. If feelings are not recognized and the information properly used or spoken about, then they may be acted out.

To recognize and talk about feelings is the response of an adult. To act upon them without thought is that of a child. For example, in the treatment of a middle-aged man with anxiety symptoms following his marriage break-up, the doctor found herself becoming increasingly irritated by the patient's reluctance to look at his own behaviour and to examine possible solutions. She was on the point of terminating the consultation when, recognizing these feelings, she brought herself to comment on them. This led to the patient being able for the first time to explore the nature of his relationships with women and of his behaviour, which so often led to his being rejected.

Our understanding of the intricacies of the doctor–patient relationship in the context of general practice has been greatly enhanced by the work of the psychiatrist and clinical teacher, Michael Balint. In a series of studies conducted with a group of general practitioners in the 1950s, he describes several important concepts which continue to be applicable to clinical practice wherever it is undertaken (Balint, 1986).

First, he regarded the continuing relationship of doctor and patient, with all its shared experiences, as being of benefit to both:

> It is not love or mutual respect or mutual identification or friendship, though elements of all these enter into it. We termed it – for want of a better term – a 'mutual investment company'. By this we mean that the general practitioner gradually acquires a valuable capital invested in his patient and, vice versa, the patient acquires a very valuable capital bestowed in his general practitioner.

While doctors learn much about their patients over the years, so the patients learn how much and what kind of help they can expect from their doctor. Balint refers to this conditioning of the patients' expectations as the 'apostolic function' of doctors, which brings us to another key concept, that of the drug, 'doctor'. He suggested that in the administration of 'themselves', doctors should be aware of their own pharmacology – whether this is as the authoritative guardian, the scientist, the protective parent, or the adviser in an equal partnership.

The changing nature of the relationship

The sociological approach to the understanding of the doctor–patient relationship is concerned with power, authority and control. The roles of doctor and patient, like other roles such as mother, husband and teacher, are associated with certain expectations that consist of both rights and obligations.

The view has been expressed that medical consultations take place in the context of a power struggle between doctor and patient, with the control of information being part of that conflict. A proponent of this view comments:

> The professional is jealous of his prerogative to diagnose and forecast illness, holding it tightly to himself. But while he does not want anyone else to give information to the patient, neither is he himself inclined to do so (Friedson, 1970).

Critics such as Illich (1976) and Kennedy (1981) have accused the medical profession of conspiring to subjugate the sick and of exploiting the public interest. However, Tuckett et al. (1985), whose research has involved the observation and analysis of over 1000 general practice consultations, challenge the view that the battle for control in the consulting room is as 'hot' as some suggest: 'Whatever the emotional difficulties, social conflicts or competence gaps, some attempt to share information is probably routine'. Thus, there is evidence to support the view that some doctors are now pursuing the goal of achieving well-informed and autonomous patients (see Chapter 2).

A number of changes are taking place in our society that should facilitate the achievement of this goal:

- The public has greater access to information on health matters through the media and the internet.
- There is an increasing emphasis on personal responsibility for health, characterized by health promotion activities.
- The economics of health are encouraging a more market-oriented approach to the provision of care. The views of the consumer are being sought through, for example, patient participation groups, which are now being set up in a number of general practices, and by national surveys of patient and user experience. (Department of Health, 1997).
- The role of the doctor as health educator is now more widely accepted (see Chapters 7 and 8).
- The need for doctors to be effective communicators has been emphasized by the General Medical Council (1993) and increasingly acknowledged by medical schools and postgraduate institutions. Indeed, communication-skills training is now an integral part of undergraduate medical curricula in almost all medical schools. (See Chapter 6).

These changes should encourage the development of the doctor–patient relationship as a partnership in care, providing that we as doctors maintain those essential elements of trust, mutual respect and empathy.

> We conceive of the consultation as a meeting between one person who has, by his training and expertise, access to scarce and specialist knowledge and another person who has, by experience, immersion in his culture and past discussion, a set of ideas about what is happening to him. Both parties form models of what is wrong, what should be done, what are the consequences of the problem, its treatment and so on, based on their own reasoning and background knowledge (Tuckett *et al.*, 1985).

The practical uses of the doctor–patient relationship

The doctor–patient relationship is not, however, merely an academic concept – it has tangible and extremely practical consequences for both doctor and patient. This is a realization that has long been recognized, as the following statement indicates.

> The significance of the intimate personal relationship between physician and patient cannot be too strongly emphasized for, in an extraordinarily large number of cases, both diagnosis and treatment depend directly upon it, and the failure of the young physician to establish this relationship accounts for much of his ineffectiveness in the care of the patient (Peabody, 1927).

Implicit in the intimacy of the consultation between doctor and patient is the confidentiality of the transaction. You will be aware, from your own experience, that intimacy is an important part of the framework of general practice, and is one characteristic that sets it apart from hospital-based medicine. Here you may wish to reflect on those other unique characteristics of primary care which nurture the doctor–patient relationship. These are discussed in detail in Chapter 1.

* Accessibility of the doctor
* Autonomy of the patient
* Personal, comprehensive and continuing care.

There are also, of course, certain characteristics in a doctor that will foster a good relationship. These include empathy, sympathy and honesty. Empathy has been described earlier as the capacity to put oneself imaginatively into someone else's position and experience the feelings which doing so arouses. Sympathy involves recognizing the other person's feelings and sharing the view that these feelings are appropriate. At the same time the doctor must, where necessary, be able to show sufficient detachment to persuade a patient to take a decision which is in the patient's best interest, yet which may not be the one the patient would choose; for example, hospital referral or admission. Another important characteristic is honesty. If both the doctor and patient feel that the communications between them are honest, frank and straightforward, the mutual trust they have is likely to grow.

How, then, can this unique relationship influence patient care? There are three main areas to consider – diagnosis, whole-person medicine and compliance.

Diagnosis

In the process of clinical reasoning discussed in Chapter 3, the importance of existing 'cues' is emphasized. By this is meant doctors' prior knowledge of their patients, which may include their attitude to illness, personality, family background and past medical history – part of the 'interest' of Balint's mutual investment company.

A good doctor–patient relationship will also encourage patients to confide more readily in their doctor. This will greatly facilitate the diagnostic process, as in the following example.

Case history
For example, Mr Brown, a 45-year-old factory worker, was seen by the new partner in the practice when the doctor he usually consulted was off duty. He complained of chest pain and, on further questioning, denied any relationship of the pain to exercise or stress. The doctor was unsure about the nature of the pain, arranged for an exercise ECG and asked Mr Brown to make a further appointment.

The following day Mr Brown returned, and was seen this time by his usual doctor. He too was unconvinced about the pain, but had known the patient for many years and was aware that he often experienced somatic symptoms when under stress. The good relationship that had developed between them enabled the doctor to utilize this information and facilitated their communication. Mr Brown, normally a diffident man, was able to confide in his doctor, who he trusted, and discuss the difficulties he was having with his foreman at work – information he had denied the new partner.

The exercise ECG was normal and Mr Brown was given appropriate reassurance and advice. In time, the work situation improved and the chest pain resolved.

Whole-person medicine

What shall we call the disease presented by a man who has always been frail, but has worked hard to support his widowed mother, did not feel he could afford to get married, buries himself in the details of a complicated job, develops paralysing headaches, loses time at the office for which pay is deducted from his wages, worries about this so much that he loses sleep and begins vomiting after each meal? (Menninger, 1956).

A clinical history almost always extends beyond the symptoms of the disease. The existence of a good doctor–patient relationship will heighten the doctor's awareness of the interplay and relative importance of social, psychological and physical factors. This allows an optimum balance to be struck between treating the illness and tailoring the management to suit the particular circumstances of the individual patient, as in the following example.

Case history
Mary consulted her doctor complaining of headaches and exhaustion. Her husband, George, had died 3 years previously, leaving her with two teenage sons and in considerable financial hardship. She is a frequent attender at the surgery with minor complaints. Finding no evidence of organic disease, the doctor encouraged her to talk – 'There was an incident a few weeks ago involving one of the boys with the police . . .'. This had confirmed her worst fears of being an inadequate parent and of failing George.

To echo Menninger, what shall we call this disease?

Compliance
It is well recognized that many patients ignore the advice of their doctor. In various studies it has been shown that an average of 50% of patients do not take their prescribed treatment or reject their doctor's advice about changes of lifestyle (Sackett, 1976; Reynolds, 1978; Ley, 1979). Failure to carry out treatment or follow advice can, of course, be due to human characteristics such as forgetfulness and procrastination, but these studies of non-compliance suggest that it is more likely to be due to inadequate or misleading information from the doctor. The provision of accurate information not only lets patients know what to do, but is also important in motivating them to do what they are advised. This applies whether the advice relates to a change of behaviour, health education or the taking of a drug. Take the example of a middle-aged businessman who comes to the doctor for an insurance medical. The doctor advises him to stop smoking, take more exercise and lose weight. He also mentions that his blood pressure is rather high and that, if it remains so after a further two readings, he will have to consider treatment. How can a man who feels well be convinced that he should change his lifestyle and take drugs which may have distressing side-effects in order to prevent an event which might, or might not, occur some time in the future? Certainly, if treatment is to be jointly planned

or negotiated, the sharing of information is necessary to help the patient retain his autonomy and to make the choices which he feels are relevant to him. A recent report from a working party of the Royal Pharmaceutical Society of Great Britain (1997) has proposed the term 'concordance' rather than 'compliance' to reflect this negotiated agreement between doctor and patient – the patient being acknowledged as a decision maker in his own treatment or care. They point out, however, that 'the price of concordance is greater responsibility – of the doctor, for the quality of the diagnosis, the treatment and the explanation; of the patient for the consequences of her or his choices' (see Chapter 8).

There is a growing body of evidence relating particular aspects of the doctor–patient interaction to effectiveness in improving health outcomes. Although mentioned earlier in Chapter 2, such evidence is worthy of reinforcement. Inui and colleagues (1976) achieved significant improvement in the control of raised blood pressure in a group of patients whose physicians had received additional training as health educators. Helping patients to learn and understand about their condition resulted in better compliance. Furthermore, in a series of studies of patients with diabetes, hypertension and peptic ulcer disease, Kaplan and colleagues (1989) have shown that more control by patients and more information sought by patients and given by the doctor are associated with better health on follow-up. This was demonstrated objectively by assessment of functional capacity and by physiological measurements.

Finally, it has been shown that the existence of a relationship where there is mutual trust, respect and effective communication is a major factor in improving compliance (Pendleton et al., 1984).

Why do some relationships go wrong?

All happy families resemble each other, each unhappy family is unhappy in its own way (from Anna Karenina, by Tolstoy).

The doctor–patient interaction, however, does not *always* lead to a satisfactory relationship. As the quotation suggests, the problems are varied and particular to each relationship. There are, however, some areas of recurrent difficulty, an awareness of which may prevent a relationship from becoming dysfunctional.

Assumptions

The doctor–patient relationship cannot be considered in isolation from other social influences, but is part of a continuum of experiences. Both doctor and patient bring to the consultation their own set of attitudes and beliefs, prejudices and expectations. These will be influenced by such factors as social class, age, ethnic origin, social and educational background and past experiences. Browne and Freeling (1976) refer to this as 'our assumptive worlds'.

The worlds of doctors and their patients may be very different, and difficulties can arise when doctors have not recognized their own assumptions or tried to understand those of their patients. The therapeutic outcome of the consultation may never reach its potential if doctors and patients do not start from the same premise about the nature of the problem and are not in agreement about the possible solution.

For example, Miss Smith, aged 24 years, came to the surgery complaining of headaches and tiredness. The doctor could find no abnormality on physical examination and told her so, asking her if she was under any stress at work or home. This she denied vehemently, saying, 'I'm not imagining it, doctor. It's not just nerves!' She would not be reassured and the doctor felt pressured into carrying out some investigations. The results were normal, but Miss Smith was still not satisfied and asked to be referred to a neurologist.

Clearly, there was no negotiation here about what was to be treated. The patient's assumptions about the nature of mental illness were not explored by the doctor, and no satisfactory explanation was given to her for her symptoms.

Consider the following: Mrs Wiseman, a well-groomed lady of 65 years, consulted the doctor about aches in the hips and knees. The doctor explained that she probably had a degree of osteoarthritis, which was part of the normal ageing process, prescribed a course of anti-inflammatory drugs and asked to see her again in a month. Mrs Wiseman never came back; she had arranged to see another partner, complaining that: 'Dr X said it was all to do with my age'.

The doctor's assumptions about the capabilities and lifestyle of the 65-year-old lady did not match those of the patient, who was still very active, playing golf twice a week, and president of the local Women's Institute. She was angry at the implication that she was 'aged'.

Detachment

It is difficult to have a close relationship with a person or family without getting involved, to some extent, with their problems. However, a degree of detachment is necessary for appropriate diagnosis and management. A balance has to be struck so that the doctor can be both caring and effective. The choice of a career of caring for people may, of course, satisfy a personal need in the carer. While there is nothing intrinsically wrong about this reciprocal situation, we need to be aware of it so that we can recognize the dangers of over-commitment. William May (1975), writing on detachment, states:

It will not do to pretend to be the second person of the Trinity, prepared to make with every patient the sympathetic descent into his suffering . . . It is important to remain emotionally free so as to be able to withdraw the self when [one's] services are no longer pertinent.

This need for a degree of detachment is particularly important when caring for the chronically sick or the dying, where the contact with patients and their families is likely to be both frequent and emotionally demanding.

Anxiety

Too close a relationship with a patient may have the effect of increasing anxiety in the problem-solving process and impairing judgement. The doctor may not feel able to tolerate uncertainty or to use time as a diagnostic tool, but instead may feel impelled to implement inappropriate referral or investigation.

For example, a doctor was consulted by the wife of one of his personal friends, complaining of vague headaches. History and examination revealed no obvious underlying cause. However, the doctor, fearing that he 'might be missing something' and reflecting on the implications this might have for his friendship, referred her to a neurologist. The neurologist was sure there was no intracranial lesion, but wondered about sinusitis. He referred the patient to an ear, nose and throat surgeon, who was unconvinced about the sinusitis but also felt obliged to investigate further. The investigations proved negative and fortunately brought to an end this example of the 'cascade' effect in clinical care, described by Mold and Stein (1986), where a single seemingly innocuous clinical characteristic initiates an unstoppable series of events resulting in more and more inappropriate medical care being offered.

The difficult patient

Since general practitioners are readily accessible to their patients and contract to undertake continuing and comprehensive care, they have to cope with those patients in whom diagnosis is not possible, who will not comply with treatment or who do not get better – the so-called 'heartsink patients' (O'Dowd, 1988).

It is widely known that a large part of the general practitioner's time is taken up with a small proportion of patients. Most of these, of course, have chronic disease or are terminally ill, but others are demanding because the relationship satisfies some need that may not be verbalized. Grol (1990), writing on this theme, uses the term 'somatic fixation'. By this he means the phenomenon which occurs when people come to depend on others, particularly health professionals, to a greater extent than is necessary, or when they become trapped in a medical maze as a result of a continuous process of inadequate reaction to illness, complaints or problems. This inability to cope or react adequately to problems can refer to the patient himself, to others in his environment, or to health care professionals.

Doctors often feel frustrated or manipulated by these patients but, as Grol suggests, may themselves contribute to the development of the behaviour. The following problems illustrate how this can occur.

Frequent attendance

These are the familiar recurring names in the appointment book, which may fill the doctor's heart with dread: those for whom no medicine is effective or who, cured of one ill, rapidly develop another. It may not be possible for even the most sensitive doctor to understand the underlying needs of this group of patients. The doctor may have to accept that a certain amount of contact is necessary and that intervention should be minimal. It is often helpful in managing this group of patients to establish a 'contract', wherein both doctor and patient agree on the frequency and conditions under which a consultation will take place.

For example, Agnes was a regular visitor to the surgery with multiple and varying complaints. From time to time the doctor would try to probe beyond the presentation or would make some minor change in medication. Agnes would always return 2 days later, with a smile on her face, saying either that the medicine hadn't worked or that she was sensitive to it. If the doctor tried to send her away without a return appointment she would be back within the week with another problem. They now have an agreement whereby Agnes makes an appointment every 4 weeks, during which time her doctor will listen to her problems and acknowledge them, but rarely attempt any active management. Both doctor and patient know where they stand. Agnes continues to function in her own way and the doctor has stopped looking at her as a failure of treatment.

Dependence

The long-term nature of the doctor–patient relationship in primary care makes this a particular problem for the general practitioner. In many instances the dependence may be temporary and the aim should be to encourage the patient towards independence, although this may not always be possible. Doctors can, however, create or contribute to dependence by seeing patients too often or by arranging unnecessary follow-up consultations and home visits. In this way doctors may satisfy a personal need in believing themselves to be indispensable. When this situation develops, the patient is at risk of losing his autonomy. According to Campbell (1984):

We feel cared for when *our* need is recognized and when the help which is offered does not overwhelm us but gently restores our strength at a pace which allows us to feel part of the movement to recovery. Conversely, a care which imposes itself on us, forcing a conformity to someone else's ideas of what we need, merely makes us feel more helpless and vulnerable.

Conclusions

Montagu (1963), in writing about the practice of clinical medicine, stated:

> Clinical medicine should be regarded neither as an art nor a science in itself, but as a special kind of relationship between two persons, a doctor and a patient.

The doctor–patient relationship, as with all other relationships, matures at its own pace. The intimacy and trust that develops quickly with one patient may take years with another. To each relationship both doctor and patient bring their own characteristics, expectations, prejudices and assumptions. It is the meeting of these two often very different worlds that can determine the nature of the relationship. This requires a willingness on the doctor's part to accept the autonomy of the patient and to be prepared to explore together any hopes and fears, so that they can come to a mutual understanding of how best to manage the problem. Writing on this theme of shared understanding, Tuckett *et al*. (1985) referred to the consultation as 'a meeting between experts'.

For the relationship to be successful and effective in terms of clinical care, doctors also require an awareness of human behaviour to understand better both patients and themselves. They must be able to communicate effectively and sensitively so that patients will be able, where appropriate, to discuss emotional, personal or family problems, yet they must remain sufficiently detached to be effective as advisers.

No consultation exists in isolation, but is part of a continuum of shared experiences from which, in time, both doctor and patient will reap 'interest'. The magnitude of such interest is directly related to the extent to which a good relationship is created and maintained between doctor and patient.

Key points

- The doctor–patient relationship is a powerful and integral component of clinical method.
- The unique characteristics of general practice – personal, comprehensive and continuing care – facilitate the development of a good doctor–patient relationship.
- The characteristics of the doctor that will encourage a good relationship to develop include sympathy, empathy and honesty.
- For the relationship to be successful and effective, doctors require an understanding of human behaviour and an awareness of their own feelings and how to use them. They must also be able to communicate effectively and sensitively with patients and their relatives.
- A good doctor–patient relationship facilitates the practice of whole-person medicine.
- A good doctor–patient relationship is a major factor in influencing compliance with treatment and advice, which can result in significant improvements in health outcomes for the patient.
- Too close a relationship may adversely affect the clinical process by increasing the doctor's anxiety, by encouraging dependency of the patient on the doctor, or by preventing the doctor from retaining a degree of appropriate emotional detachment.

References

Balint, M. (1986). *The Doctor, His Patient and The Illness*, 3rd edn. Edinburgh: Churchill Livingstone.

Berne, E. (1973). *Games People Play*. London: Penguin.

Brown, D. and Pedder, J. (1979). *Introduction to Psychotherapy*, pp. 58–66. London: Tavistock Publications.

Browne, K. and Freeling, P. (1976). *The Doctor–Patient Relationship*, 2nd edn, pp. 14–19, 58–64. Edinburgh: Churchill Livingstone.

Campbell, A. V. (1984). *Moderated Love. A Theology of Professional Care*, pp. 107–8. London: SPCK.

Department of Health for England (1997). *The New NHS*. London: The Stationery Office Ltd.

Federman, D. D. (1990). The education of medical students: sounds, alarums and excursions. *Academic Medicine*, 65(4), 221–6.

Friedson, E. (1970). *Professional Dominance*. Chicago: Atherton Press.

General Medical Council (1993). *Tomorrow's Doctors. Recommendations on Undergraduate Medical Education*. London: General Medical Council.

Grol, R. (1990). *To Heal or to Harm. The Prevention of Somatic Fixation in General Practice*. London: Royal College of General Practitioners.

Illich, I. (1976). *Limits to Medicine. Medical Nemesis: The Expropriation of Health*. London: Maryon Boyards.

Inui, T. S., Yourtree, F. L. and Williamson, I. W. (1976). Improved outcomes in hypertension after physician tutorials. A controlled trial. *Annals of Internal Medicine*, 84, 646.

Kaplan, S. H., Greenfield, S. and Ware I. F. (1989). Assessing the effects of patient–physician interactions on the outcomes of chronic disease. *Medical Care*, 27, Silo.

Kennedy, I. (1981). *The Unmasking of Medicine*. London: George Allen and Unwin.

Ley, P. (1979). Memory for medical information. *British Journal of the Society of Clinical Psychology*, **18**, 245.

May, W. F. (1975). Code, covenant, contract or philanthropy. *The Hastings Center Report*, **5**, 30.

Menninger, W. C. (1956). Psychiatry and the practice of medicine. *Mississippi Valley Medical Journal*.

Mold, J. W. and Stein H. F. (1986). The cascade effect in the clinical care of patients. *New England Medical Journal*, **314**, 512–14.

Montagu, A. (1963). Anthropology and medical education. *Journal of the American Medical Association*, **183**, 577.

O'Dowd, T. C. (1988). Five years of heartsink patients in general practice. *British Medical Journal*, **297**, 528.

Peabody, F. (1927). The care of the patient. *Journal of the American Medical Association*, **88**, 877.

Pendleton, D., Tate, P., Havelock, P. and Schofield T. (1984). *The Consultation: An Approach to Learning and Teaching*. Oxford: Oxford University Press.

Reynolds, M. (1978). No news is bad news: patients' views about communication in hospital. *British Medical Journal*, **1**, 1973.

Royal Pharmaceutical Society of Great Britain (1997). *From Compliance to Concordance: Towards Shared Goals in Medicine Taking*. London: RPS.

Sackett, D. L. (1976). Introduction. In *Compliance with Therapeutic Regimens* (D. L. Sackett and R. B. Haynes, eds.). Baltimore: Johns Hopkins University Press.

Tuckett, D., Boulton, M., Olsen, C. and Williams, A. (1985). *Meetings Between Experts*. London: Tavistock Publications.

6
Doctor–patient communication

M. Elan Preston-Whyte

> . . . problems with doctor–patient
> communication are extremely common and
> adversely affect patient management. It has
> been repeatedly shown that the clinical skills
> needed to improve these problems can be
> taught and that the subsequent benefits to
> medical practice are demonstrable . . . and
> enduring (Simpson *et al.*, 1991).

This chapter will examine why doctors must be good communicators if
they are to practise effectively. It will also highlight those skills which a
doctor needs to acquire in order to accomplish those tasks of the
consultation which relate particularly to communications between doctor
and patient. These have already been explicitly described in Chapter 2.

The quotations used in this chapter have been chosen to illustrate
points in the text. They have been taken from two main sources:
unpublished extracts from tape-recorded experiences of patients in
general practice made by a sociologist researcher in the Department of
Community Health, University of Leicester (K. Dodd, 1980) and from an
essay written by a second year Leicester medical student (N. Russell,
1984). Although women patients do consult more frequently than men it
is purely fortuitous that the majority of the quotations are from women
patients. The opinions expressed are from across the whole range of
social class, and span an age range from 21 to 83 years.

Why doctors must be good communicators

The diagnosis of a condition and an understanding of its effects on a
patient's life and experience clearly depend on the doctor creating the
conditions in which the patient can accurately transmit a message and
the doctor can accurately receive that message. The doctor can do this
by using particular verbal and non-verbal behaviour to enable a patient
to talk freely; also by correctly interpreting the signals the patient is
sending out and by relaying back to the patient that the message is

received and understood. This lays the foundation of the history taking process, which is the key to the consultation (see Chapter 3), although communication skills are also deployed during physical examinations.

Good communication also helps to establish a relationship between the doctor and patient, which has an important and beneficial effect on the outcome of the consultation. Patients who think that they have been allowed to tell the doctor what they feel is relevant about their problem, who have had the problem interpreted in language that they can understand and who have been given advice that is simple and appropriate, will be far more likely to comply with that advice than patients who have not been dealt with in this way (McWhinney, 1989). An 83-year-old widow had this to say about her doctor:

> He was very attentive – well, he was with me. He'd sit and listen and say 'Well, come on, tell me all about it'. And he'd sit there and you'd pour out all your troubles and he'd listen like a father. And I loved him for that, you know, because I thought to myself, well, he's real interested.

Consider, however, the comments of a printer's wife, aged 30 years:

> You could count the time I was in with him in seconds, because he'd got your medical card there and when you walked in your name was already on the prescription . . . and he's signed it. He'd be writing it out as you were talking.

Because communication between individuals is part of everyday life it is often assumed, by both medical teachers and students, that all that is required to communicate with patients is the intuitive application of the same skills as those required in social settings (Royston, 1997). Not all individuals possess them to the same degree, however, nor can they use them with equal effect. However, they can be learnt or developed (see Appendices 1 and 2 to this chapter) in the same way as more traditional medical skills such as performing a lumbar puncture or taking a blood pressure (Fallowfield, 1996; Roter *et al.*, 1990, 1998).

Maguire and Rutter (1976) have demonstrated that the traditional apprenticeship method of training medical students to take histories often fails to teach them sufficient interviewing skills to enable them to obtain a full and accurate account of their patients' problems. They also showed that students can acquire these skills, however, particularly through feedback training. Furthermore, when followed up 5 years later these former students, when compared with their contemporaries who had not received such training, were better in the skills associated with accurate diagnosis.

In real life it is hard for doctors to receive critical feedback on their behaviour, because dissatisfied patients do not usually tell the doctor that they feel that way. They more often demonstrate it by not returning to the doctor, who may remain completely unaware of the reason for their absence, thereby removing a stimulus to self-improvement.

The communication skills needed in the consultation

The consultation consists of two distinct parts: the *interview*, in which the doctor seeks to discover why a patient has come to seek help, and the *exposition*, in which the doctor informs the patient of any findings (including diagnosis) and discusses with the patient the treatment and advice considered needed. From the point of view of doctor–patient communication, Brown (1978) has identified the key skills of the consultation as follows:

Questioning
Listening
Responding
Explaining.

The skills required in the two parts of the consultation are in many ways distinct. In the interview the skills of questioning, listening and responding are particularly important, whilst explaining is a skill which should be used sparingly. When the exposition is reached, however, explaining is the skill which is paramount, together with negotiating and collaborating skills (see also Chapter 4 on Patient Management).

The interview

The opening

Patients are often anxious about coming to see doctors. The following quotation graphically illustrates how a patient felt as she sat waiting her turn:

> I think when you go and see the doctor, well I do . . . you go and you think, especially if you don't feel well, and you don't know how to explain to the doctor what's wrong. You sit in the waiting room with all those things going round in your mind; where shall I start, what shall I say first, how can I explain how I feel? . . . I get all panicky inside . . . (Tuckett *et al.*, 1985).

Patient anxiety can be alleviated in several ways, and the opening of the consultation is the key to putting patients at ease. Korsch and Negrete (1972) found that the friendliness of the doctor correlates well with the satisfaction of patients with the consultation. The doctor can communicate this to patients in various ways, e.g. greeting patients by name, rising to meet them, shaking their hand, indicating where they can sit and engaging in some preliminary informal chat. These are all verbal and non-verbal behaviours that will help to diminish or eliminate the natural anxiety experienced by most patients early in the consultation.

A van driver's wife, aged 34 years, praised her doctor because:

> As soon as you walked in, he'd always got a smile on his face. He just put you at ease as soon as you sat down.

In contrast, a roof-tiler's wife, aged 22 years, commented about her experience:

> You'd sit down in front of his desk and usually he'd be writing something and you'd just sit down and wait until he looked up . . .

In general practice, other factors have been identified which influence patient satisfaction with their doctors: patients rate highly the opportunity to see the same doctor over a period of time, that is, they value personal care and continuity of care. Other characteristics such as the sex and age of the doctor appear to have less influence on satisfaction (Baker, 1996), although patients may prefer to consult a doctor of the same sex for potentially embarrassing problems (Preston-Whyte et al., 1983).

The setting of the consultation can strongly influence the type of communication that will take place, and is to a large extent under the control of the doctor. This will include the appearance (i.e. dress and grooming) of the doctor and the seating arrangement of doctor and patient (see Figure 6.1). The side-by-side position is regarded as aiding co-operation, directly-facing positions are seen as confronting, while sitting at a 90° angle is associated with friendly conversation (Argyle, 1983).

Doctors may manipulate the relative orientation of themselves and their patients by leaving patients with no choice as to where they may sit. When a choice is allowed, the exercise of that choice by patients may reveal a great deal of their personality – those who are shy will usually prefer to sit further away to protect their personal space.

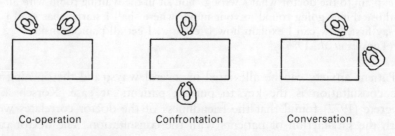

Co-operation   Confrontation   Conversation

Figure 6.1   Seating arrangements of doctor and patient

The history

The welcome over, the doctor then indicates that the patient should begin to relate the problem. The doctor may do this with a noncommittal 'Well, now?' or, more specifically, 'What can I do for you?' – either opening giving the patient a choice in the way to respond. The objective of the initial part of the interview is to encourage and enable patients to give their story as fully as possible in their own words.

The appearance of the doctor, i.e. dress (formal or casual) and grooming (neat and tidy, grubby or dishevelled), will already have met or not met the patient's expectations of the doctor's role. The posture adopted will influence the transaction even more; leaning forward facing the patient, nearness, touching and gaze signal intimacy and liking. An atmosphere of warmth and empathy is encouraged – sometimes touching the patient may appropriately convey concern when the patient is distressed. A 25-year-old unmarried mother of two obviously felt keenly what she perceived to be a lack of interest shown by her doctor when she said:

> He's never touched me – never. It's just a matter of interest. I mean, even if you don't like someone, you can touch them. There's no harm in that, is there?

Questioning and listening

The doctor may find it helpful, once the major problems appear to have
• been stated, to summarize what the patient has related in order to confirm that the doctor's perception of the information given matches that of the patient. If not, further clarification is required.

The doctor can now employ various types of questions in the search for particular pieces of information that may suggest certain diagnoses or facilitate a deeper exploration of the patient's problem.

Open questions encourage patients to reveal information that might not otherwise have been volunteered, e.g. 'Tell me how the problem has affected you.' Patients' answers may provide insights into their physical or emotional state that may suggest a new line of questioning. The disadvantage of the open question, however, is that it encourages patients to talk more, which may result in the doctor being overwhelmed with information, some of which may be irrelevant. As a consequence the interview may be more difficult for the doctor to control – a particular problem for students (Maguire and Rutter, 1976), who may feel that patients would consider it rude to be interrupted. A strategy to adopt may be to interrupt politely and say to the patient 'this information (observation) is interesting, but I need to focus on particular areas to try and solve your problem'. This provides the student with the opportunity to guide the consultation to more fruitful areas of enquiry.

Probing questions may now be more useful. These are follow-up questions that stimulate patients to think more deeply about their answers. For instance, if a patient's presenting problem was pain, the doctor could ask: 'Have you noticed anything which brings on the pain?'

Prompts are questions that contain hints to encourage patients to augment their story. For instance, the doctor might ask: 'You say the pain comes on when you move. Can you describe more precisely what movement brings it on?'

Closed questions are likely to produce only short answers, usually yes or no options, and are useful when the doctor is searching for particular items of information to confirm or refute likely diagnoses. The advantage of closed questions is that they save time and can be used quite legitimately by the doctor in certain circumstances. For instance, if a doctor wishes to test a theory that a patient's vague symptomatology could be due to a malignancy somewhere, supporting evidence may be sought by asking 'Have you lost weight?' or 'Have you coughed up any blood?' The disadvantages of closed questions are that they provide limited information, falsification is easy and their inappropriate use frustrates and irritates patients, who feel they need more opportunity to explain. Because the inductive type of history taking uses mainly closed questions, students tend to over-use them out of habit.

Leading questions are best avoided, because they encourage patients to give answers they think the doctor might like to hear. For example, if the doctor asks 'Would you agree that this pain could be due to anxiety?', patients are likely to concur even though it may not reflect their true feelings. The question would be better phrased as follows: 'Sometimes a pain like this can be made worse by anxiety, could this be possible in your case?' This gives patients more opportunity to qualify their answer as necessary.

Pausing *before* and *after* asking a difficult question ensures that patients understand what is implied. Additionally, the doctor may forewarn the patient by prefacing the question with 'My next question may not be an easy one for you to answer, so I will give you time to think about your response'.

Double-barrelled questions, i.e. asking patients two overlapping questions, should also be avoided because patients may be confused as a result and be unable to reply accurately to both. For instance, 'Have you tried taking paracetamol . . . or an antacid for your pain?' may result in the patient replying 'yes', but the doctor will not know to which drug this answer applies. A better approach would be to ask two separate questions or an open question, such as 'Have you taken anything for the pain?'.

While bearing in mind that the interview should be patient-centred, the doctor still needs to maintain the right degree of control in consultations. In the interview phase, summarizing what has been said at certain stages and politely negotiating with the patient what areas to cover next will help to bring the patient back to the point.

Another mistake that students make – usually because of their anxiety to formulate the next question – is not to listen to the reply the patient has given to their previous question; a condition aptly described as 'What shall I say the next time the patient inhales?' (Bendix, 1982). This brings us to the skill of *listening*, which is all-important throughout the consultation. This does not mean just sitting passively until the patient 'runs out of steam', but involves attempting to understand the message the patient is trying to convey, both verbally and non-verbally. Patients can readily recognize when a doctor is actively listening and giving them full attention by the doctor's posture and demeanour. A 52-year-old engineer recognized his doctor as a poor listener:

> The previous GP was lousy . . . he was not the listening type. You could see it going through that side and coming out this side (pointing to his head) . . . It was difficult to communicate.

In order to listen, doctors need to be relaxed but vigilant. They should be aware of the possible distractions which may affect their ability to hear and understand what the patient is saying – for example, a restless child accompanying a patient, phone calls or reception staff interrupting the consultation, looking at the patient's records for past information, etc. Video recordings of consultations are invaluable sources of self-feedback on performance because they may reveal that the patient has mentioned some essential fact or hinted at a possible area of concern that the doctor had completely missed. (See also Chapter 11).

It is also important not to interrupt the patient's narrative, particularly in the early stages of the interview. If, however, it contains items to which the doctor wishes to return, writing key words or phrases as an *aide-memoire* to questions that can be asked at a more appropriate time is useful. It is not advisable to take extensive notes as the patient speaks because this inevitably interferes with the ability to listen to and observe the patient closely; behaviour that will not only be noticed by the patient, but will also exert a negative impact.

When it is necessary to interrupt, however, for instance when the patient begins to repeat information already given, then this should be done sensitively and politely by saying, 'What you have told me has been very helpful, but I would now like you to focus on . . .'.

Non-verbal behaviour

Throughout interviews, doctors should be self-aware – i.e. noticing the effect of their behaviour on the patient and vice versa. What clues are there in the sort of language patients use to tell their story, or the emotion with which they invest it? Observation and analysis of a patient's non-verbal behaviour is particularly important, as the doctor can glean much information from it concerning the personality and attitude of the patient (Argyle, 1975). Indeed, the impact of words is often weaker and less direct than the impact of non-verbal signals. It is well-recognized that words do not always convey the truth. Consequently, the doctor should be prepared to place a considerable degree of dependence on non-verbal cues, since they are less easily controlled by the patient and may therefore be a more genuine indication of how the patient really feels.

Movements of the mouth, eyes and eyebrows are most expressive of a variety of emotions, while skin colour may indicate anxiety (white) or anger (flushed). The amount of eye contact made by a patient and the degree of pupil dilatation can also be revealing. Patients who avoid your gaze may do so because of shyness or embarrassment, or because they are not telling the truth. Pupil dilatation occurs when a patient is extremely anxious or has a strong feeling of affiliation towards the doctor. Gestures add vividly to the words accompanying them, since jerking or tapping movements of the feet or fingers often reveal an inner tension. The patient's posture should be observed to see whether it is tense or relaxed; for example, tension may be indicated by the patient sitting stiffly or moving restlessly.

Responding

Doctors should respond to any observed emotional signals by indicating that they recognize their importance to the patient. They can do this by using encouraging nods and gestures and by touching the patient as and when appropriate. It may be necessary to confront a patient directly with the effect that the story is producing. In this context, confrontation does not involve a threatening or aggressive manner, as is commonly understood by the word. It is a technique whereby doctors can use the emotion generated in a consultation in a constructive manner to make the patient more aware of its implications. For example, a depressed patient may not readily admit to being depressed but may generate a profound feeling of depression in the doctor. The doctor can reflect this emotion back to the patient by saying, 'What you have told me and the way in which you have told it makes me feel rather depressed – how do you feel about it?'

Patients are usually willing to let doctors explore potentially embarrassing or emotionally distressing areas in their histories if they are made aware of the relevance that this exploration may have to the diagnosis and possible solution of their problems. Doctors need to be able to probe embarrassing areas, for instance sexual functioning and orientation, without embarrassment on their part and with sensitivity. Observing experienced doctors conducting consultations of this nature may not provide students with enough confidence to feel competent to experiment with real patients, and role play is a useful teaching method which can be employed (Baraitser *et al.*, 1998).

Reasons why the interview may fail

In the course of training medical students to communicate better, Maguire and Rutter (1976) have identified the commonest reasons for the failure of students to obtain enough relevant information from the interview. They are:

1. Failure to prepare the patient, i.e. failing to put the patient at ease before rushing to ask questions about the main complaint.
2. Failure to control the interview, i.e. allowing the patient to talk at length about matters quite unrelated to their present problems. Students did not appear to know how or when to interrupt, or how to redirect the patient's narrative to more relevant topics, because they were afraid that any attempt to interrupt or redirect the conversation might make patients unco-operative and resentful.
3. The influence of a premature or restricted focus on students, i.e. students assumed that patients have only one main problem and that this was much more likely to be organic than psychological or social in nature. Students explained that their reluctance to touch on more personal areas of enquiry was due to their anxiety that patients might find such questions unacceptable or intrusive.
4. A lack of a systematic interview procedure. This is not the same as a routine system review as used in hospital, but implies following a logical sequence of questions (as in a flow diagram) when investigating a possible diagnosis or hypothesis.
5. Lack of clarification of the information in order to establish the accuracy of the data. The uncertainty of much of the information was also due to the students' failure to detect or confront patients with obvious inconsistencies in their account. Similarly, few students made any attempt to encourage patients to date their experiences accurately.
6. Unresponsiveness to verbal and non-verbal cues. This was most noticeable when patients gave cues suggestive of emotional upset. Students intimated that they feared that if they responded to such cues they would precipitate even more distress, which they felt ill-prepared to deal with.
7. Lack of self-awareness. The students displayed mannerisms that seriously hampered their attempts to relate to their patients.
8. Difficulties with taking notes and maintaining eye contact.

It should be noted that several of these deficiencies cover ground beyond communication problems. They relate to wider consultation competences, knowledge deficits, lack of reasoning skills and relationship difficulties (see also Chapter 11).

The physical examination

Communication also takes place during the physical examination carried out by the doctor. Prior to the examination, the doctor needs to explain to the patient why an examination is required, what areas of the body this will involve and to seek the patient's explicit consent, particularly if this is to include an intimate examination. In the latter case, the doctor needs to describe what a pelvic or rectal examination will entail, including how this will be done.

Whilst students should complete their history taking before proceeding to physical examination, the act of touching the patient may facilitate a more intimate enquiry about physical symptoms, e.g. sexual functioning, which the patient may have had difficulty in mentioning before. For example, in the case of an area manager's wife, aged 28 years:

> I had problems with my marriage, the sexual side. I must have been going to Dr. X for 3 months before I finally got round to the real reason. I remember the first time I mentioned it, I felt so embarrassed, but he put me so much at my ease.

A vaginal or rectal examination should be performed as sensitively and as gently as possible. Sometimes such an examination, especially a vaginal examination, will reveal a great deal about a patient's attitude towards her sexuality and may give important clues about her sexual relationship that may not be evident from her history.

By the end of the interview and examination phases of the consultation the doctor will normally have formulated the patient's problem or problems, and the management or exposition phase of the consultation begins.

The exposition

> Good explanations, like good bikinis, should be brief, appealing, yet cover the essential features (Brown, 1978).

In the interview, explaining is a skill which should be used only in response to patients' answers or comments as there may be a temptation to explain (perhaps wrongly) too much too early. In the exposition, however, the skills of explaining employed by the doctor in communicating findings to the patient are of the essence. No matter how perceptive the diagnosis made, if the doctor is unable to explain what this means to the patient in terms that can be clearly understood the result will be a dissatisfied or confused patient who is unlikely to comply with the suggested management plan. For example:

> E took her 10-year-old son to see the GP about a lump on the side of his head just in front of his ear. The diagnosis had been 'glands', which didn't impress E as she 'didn't think you had "glands" there!'.

Throughout the exposition phase of the consultation, the doctor's thoughts and actions should be governed by the need to:

- Create the appropriate balance of priorities between the person and the illness
- Convey to the patient sympathy, empathy and honesty
- Remain aware of a patient's right to share in the decision-making process about management plans.

Furthermore, patients often have ideas about their health which may be important and relevant, and which the doctor must take into consideration in negotiating a management plan with the patient; that is, sharing of information should go in both directions. It is important for the doctor to discover, once the patient has understood the treatment options, whether the patient wishes to take responsibility for choosing a preferred option or wants the doctor to make the decision, or whether both parties should come to a shared agreement on the option to be chosen (Charles, 1997). If this approach had been heeded, then the following outcome of a consultation could have been avoided:

E had consulted the GP with a bad headache and ended up with a prescription for codydramol, sleeping pills, coproxamol and Valium – which she shouldn't have had since she once took an overdose. All she had wanted was a chat.

As patients become better educated and more aware of their rights, doctors should also be prepared for some patients to question their advice (Towle, 1998). This should be viewed as a need for further clarification rather than an assault on the doctor's judgement.

The doctor should plan his explanation as follows: first identify the problem to be explained, then ascertain the level of awareness of the patient and, finally, structure the explanation accordingly. The doctor needs to acquire verbal skills that will enable the use words readily understood by the patient. The importance of not using jargon can be seen from the following quotation from a machinist, aged 21 years:

But if ever I've been down the hospital, and they talk . . . they have a different language. And some of the terms you don't understand. And I always go to my GP if I didn't understand and ask him . . . take the medical terms with me, remember them. And he would sit and talk them out with me, and tell me what I didn't understand, the medical terms. He'd tell me all the ins and outs – he was very good.

The setting for the exposition is important. The patient should be invited to sit; if the doctor begins the summary with the patient still occupied in dressing then much of what is said will go unheard and will, therefore, not be understood or remembered.

Pendleton *et al.* (1984) have shown that patients remember well what they have been told immediately a consultation is over, but this does not mean that they have understood the message. In certain circumstances, it may be appropriate for the doctor to check the patient has understood the advice given by asking the patient to recall the essential points before leaving.

The doctor should thus summarize the findings, using the appropriate lay terms and employing verbal and graphic illustrations where these would be helpful. The reassuring aspects of the diagnosis and prognosis should be emphasized to the patient if appropriate. In circumstances where there is a great deal of information to impart, it may be necessary for the doctor to preface remarks by 'explicit categorization'. This means indicating to the patient the sort of information about to be heard. For instance,

> First, I am going to tell you what is wrong with you, then what tests will be needed, then what treatment I would advise, how you will get on and what you will have to do to help yourself . . . and finally what I would advise you to do.

The doctor should avoid giving too much information too quickly, and should place first the most critical information as this will be remembered best. A 32-year-old tool-maker was able to recall:

> The doctor explained I had an infection, and the infection had left some deposit on the windpipe that caused an irritation, which makes me cough. That was a good explanation and I understood it quite fully, and it made me happier. I know what it was all about. Instead of 'You've got a chest infection' and give you a few pills and that was it.

One of the key areas in the management of a patient is to make sure that medicines are taken in the right dose, at the right times, by the right route and in the right way (Consumer's Association, 1991). Patients can be helped to comply with the instructions on how medicines should be taken if the doctor ensures that the patient understands what advantages the treatment will confer, the important or common adverse effects that may be experienced, and what to do if the latter occurs. Patients should have ample opportunity to ask questions and, at review, should be encouraged to discuss any adverse effects. Doctors may help recollection of advice given by providing patients with information leaflets or by inviting them to record the instructions themselves. Good information material must explain the choices, enhance patients' confidence and sense of control, suggest things that might be further discussed with the doctor and help patients to identify their treatment preferences (Coulter, 1997).

An ex-army major, aged 57 years, expressed his satisfaction with his doctor's approach:

> She was my ideal doctor, and I've met many in my experience. She always had time. She didn't waste time but she always had time to talk sensibly to you and, I think, to reassure you and to find out what was wrong. She knew pretty well what was the matter with you and I think that one had tremendous confidence in her judgement. And, you know, if she was prescribing treatment or things like that, she would more or less tell you what the object of the exercise was, what it would *help* so that you felt it *would*. And I think psychologically that's important.

Breaking bad news

Breaking bad news to patients with serious or lethal diseases calls for communication skills of the highest order. Empathy, sensitivity and clear use of language will help the communication process. Furthermore, the doctor needs to develop the ability to cope with the emotional distress that the patient will almost certainly be exhibiting and the doctor will be feeling (Tattersall and Ellis, 1998; Metcalfe, 1998).

The principles of giving a patient bad news are as follows:

- Choose the right moment to tell. This may involve assessing whether the patient is receptive and feeling well enough to talk. The presence of a relative may be helpful.
- Choose a setting that is private, and where the interview will not be disturbed.
- Make sufficient time available and look unhurried.
- Proceed at the patient's pace and follow the patient's agenda in order to help the assimilation of information. This will involve exploring the patient's understanding of the situation and feelings about what has occurred and what might occur.
- Assess how much the patient knows and wants to know. The doctor can then build gradually on this knowledge by sharing information in small packages and reassessing the patient's understanding and feelings at each stage before deciding to progress.
- Identify the main concerns of the patient; potential solutions can then be discussed whilst positive areas should be emphasized to help maintain realistic hope.
- Finally, offer the patient continuing support, indicating that you are prepared to enter into a continuing relationship.

These steps are essential if the interview is to be one in which the patient can leave still trusting the doctor's integrity, yet comforted by the doctor's concern.

A patient, writing about the way in which she was told about her anal cancer, said:

> Smiles deceived, reassurances deluded, suspicions were not shared . . . the deceit hurt (Blennerhassett, 1998).

It is important that learning the skills to break bad news effectively is not left to on-the-job experience, where the learner may develop habits of survival rather than the appropriate skills, (Harden, 1996; Royston,1997). The use of actors in video-recorded consultations where the challenge is to break bad news, and where doctors receive feedback on their performance from a small group of peers and an experienced tutor, provides a safe environment for acquisition of the necessary skills (Preston-Whyte *et al.*, 1995).

Another difficult area which may be associated with breaking bad news of the sudden or unexpected death of patients is coping with the relatives grief whilst needing to make a request for organs for transplantation. Before discussing the latter issue, it is 'extremely important that relatives are given appropriate and understandable information about their loved one's condition . . . . Establishing a trusting and understanding relationship is a prerequisite to making a request for organs. If this is not the case, a refusal is most likely' (Randhawa, 1998).

The ending

The conclusion of the consultation should be as relaxed and unhurried as the opening, as exemplified by the following comments made by a town planner's wife, aged 33 years:

> She's always very chatty and it's almost like the old GP type of atmosphere. When you leave she'll always say . . . I don't know what she says really . . . something like, 'I hope you are alright' or 'Come back again'. It's more like a social chat we're having, rather than a short, sharp interview.

The objective is to assess whether patients are satisfied with what has gone before and are ready to take their leave. Clues to dissatisfaction will include hesitation in their speech, lack of eye contact and a reluctance to leave. Satisfaction is usually expressed by a positive response, such as a smile and a readiness to rise and say 'goodbye' when the doctor asks directly 'Are you happy with this?'.

Occasionally, and even when the consultation has been a long one where the doctor may feel all the relevant ground has been covered, the patient may hesitate on rising or, on reaching the door, may turn and say 'Oh, by the way, doctor . . .'. *This is a signal which should never be ignored*, because it may indicate the real reason for the consultation: all that has gone before may merely have been the 'ticket of admission' (McWhinney, 1981).

The strategies for coping with this eventuality vary with the circumstances, but the doctor should encourage the patient to proceed with whatever needs to be said. It may be necessary to invite the patient to sit down again and to explore the issue raised more fully at this time. An alternative strategy is to suggest, once the nature of the problem has been identified, that if the patient is agreeable it could be left to be dealt with at a further and, if necessary, longer consultation.

Reasons why the exposition may fail

The following are the commonest reasons for the failure of the doctor to perform effectively in the exposition:

● The doctor leaves insufficient time at the end of the consultation either to explain fully or to check that the patient has understood what has been said.
● The doctor fails to recognize and alleviate the patient's anxiety. In turn, this will impair the patient's ability to concentrate on under-standing and remembering what has been said.
● The doctor does not use explicit categorization sufficiently to prepare patients to receive large amounts of information.
● The doctor ignores the verbal and non-verbal signals from the patient that indicate that the patient is not satisfied with the explanation.
● The doctor fails to seek the patient's agreement with the proposed management of the problem, with the result that the patient does not comply with the advice given.

Maguire *et al.* (1986), in a follow-up investigation of young doctors who had received feedback on their interviewing skills as students, found that whilst their level of interviewing skill had been maintained, most remained incapable of giving patients information and advice about their problems. He related this to the lack of training they had received as students in this important aspect of clinical practice.

The following quotation illustrates how the outcome of a consultation in which doctor and patient have failed to communicate may have both immediate and longer-term repercussions:

> E said she had heard of a pill which would stop bedwetting, but when she suggested it to the GP he said he couldn't give her any but could refer the boys to a psychiatrist. E was furious at this; all she wanted was dry sheets, not psychiatry. E now says she has no faith in doctors, since none of them know what they are talking about.

The consensus statement that emerged from the 1991 Toronto Conference on doctor–patient communication ended with the following succinct conclusion:

There is . . . a clear and urgent need for teaching of these clinical skills [of doctor–patient communication] to be incorporated into medical school curricula and continued into postgraduate training (Simpson *et al.*, 1991).

Following on from the consensus statement, a working group convened at Conferences on Teaching and Assessing Communication Skills in Medical Education (Oxford, 1996, Amsterdam, 1998: personal communication) have produced the following recommendations:

- Teaching and assessment should be based on a broad view of communication in medicine.
- Communication skills teaching and clinical teaching should not be considered separately.
- There should be a planned and coherent curriculum for communication skills teaching.
- Teaching should define and help students achieve essential communication skills.
- Students' ability to achieve communication tasks should be assessed directly.
- Both teaching and assessment should foster students' personal and professional growth.
- Communication skills teaching and assessment programmes should be evaluated.
- Communication skills faculty should receive support and development as teachers.

Prescribing communication skills development for undergraduates should be only the first step, however, of a continuing medical education programme for doctors at all levels and in all disciplines. To this end, 'medical teachers have to take a leadership role in opening up channels of better communication between physicians and patients' (Meryn, 1998).

Key points

- Communication in the consultation requires the following skills, which can all be learnt and developed:
  - questioning
  - listening
  - responding
  - explaining
  - negotiating
  - reinforcing.
- Useful *tactics* for students to employ in the consultation are:
  - building on the answer obtained to a question by asking related questions at the same level
  - clarifying the problem
  - summarizing the response
  - checking back with the patient for understanding and consent.
- Good communication
  - is the basis of good history taking and hence clinical competence
  - favourably influences the quality of the doctor–patient relationship and patient compliance
  - is sensitive to the needs of patients and relatives
  - is clear, unequivocal and persuasive.

References

Argyle, M. (1975). *Bodily Communication*, Chapter 19. London: Methuen.

Argyle, M. (1983). *The Psychology of Interpersonal Behaviour*, Chapters 1–3. London: Penguin.

Baker, R. (1996). Characteristics of practices, general practitioners and patients related to levels of patients' satisfaction with consultations. *British Journal of General Practice*, 46, 601–5.

Baraitser, P., Elliott, L. and Bigsrigg, A. (1998). How to talk about sex and do it well: a course for medical students. *Medical Teacher*, 20, 237–40.

Bendix, T. (1982). Seven wrong thoughts which prevent you from behaving properly. In *The Anxious Patient. The Therapeutic Dialogue in Clinical Practice* (H. J. Wright, ed.), Chapter 2. Edinburgh: Churchill Livingstone. (A slim book which gives valuable rules of thumb on how to act, and how not to act, in consultations which have a major emotional component.)

Blennerhassett, M. (1998). Deadly charades. *British Medical Journal*, 316, 1890–91.

Brown, G. A. (1978). Exposition and listening. Questioning and answering. In *Microteaching: A Programme of Teaching Skills*, Units V and VI. London: Methuen.

Charles, C. (1997). *Shared Decision-Making in the Medical Encounter: What Does it Mean? Promoting Patient Choice Together* (a report of an international conference). London: King's Fund.

Consumer's Association (1991). Helping patients to make the best use of medicines. *Drug and Therapeutics Bulletin*, 29(1), 1.

Coulter, A. (1997). *Evidence-Based Patient Choice. Promoting Patient Choice Together* (a report of an international conference). London: King's Fund.

Fallowfield, L. J. (1996). Things to consider when teaching doctors how to deliver good, bad and sad news. *Medical Teacher*, 18, 27–30.

Harden, R. M. (1996). Twelve tips on teaching and learning how to break bad news. *Medical Teacher*, **18**(4), 275–8.

Korsch, B. M. and Negrete, V. F. (1972). Doctor–patient communication. *Scientific American*, **227**, 66–8.

McWhinney, I. R. (1981). The doctor–patient relationship. In *An Introduction to Family Medicine*. New York, Oxford: Oxford University Press.

McWhinney, I. R. (1989). The need for a transformed clinical method. In *Communicating with Medical Patients* (M. Stewart and D. Roter, eds.), pp. 25–42. Newbury Park, CA: Sage.

Maguire, P. and Rutter, D. R. (1976). History taking for medical students. 1. Deficiencies in performance. *Lancet*, **ii**, 356–8.

Maguire, P., Fairbairn, S. and Fletcher, C. (1986) Consultation skills of young doctors: I. Benefits of feedback training in interviewing as students persist. II. Most young doctors are bad at giving information. *British Medical Journal*, **292**, 1573–8.

Meryn, S. (1998). Improving communication skills: to carry coals to Newcastle. *Medical Teacher*, **20**(4), 331–6.

Metcalfe, D. (1998). Doctors and patients should be fellow travellers. *British Medical Journal*, **316**, 1892–3.

Pendleton, D. A., Schofield, T., Tate, P. and Havelock, P. (1984). *The Consultation: An Approach to Learning and Teaching*, pp. 20–22, 40–49. Oxford: Oxford University Press.

Preston-Whyte, M. E., Fraser, R. C. and Beckett, J. L. (1983). Effect of a principal's gender on consultation patterns. *British Journal of General Practice*, **33**, 654–8.

Preston-Whyte, M. E., Hastings, A. M. H. and Fraser, R. C. (1995). Breaking bad news: a workshop to enhance the skills of junior doctors. *Education for General Practice*, **6**, 306–14.

Randhawa, G. (1998). Coping with grieving relatives and making a request for organs: principles for staff training. *Medical Teacher*, **20**(3), 247–9.

Roter, D. L., Cole, K. A., Kern, D. E. *et al.* (1990). An evaluation of residency training in interviewing skills and the psychosocial domain of medical practice. *Journal of General Internal Medicine*, **5**, 347–454.

Roter, D., Rosenbaum, J., de Negri, B. *et al.* (1998). The effects of a continuing medical education programme in interpersonal communication skills on doctor practice and patient satisfaction in Trinidad and Tobago. *Medical Education*, **32**, 181–9.

Royston, V. (1997). How do medical students learn to communicate with patients? A study of fourth-year medical students' attitudes to doctor–patient communication. *Medical Teacher*, **19**(4), 257–62.

Simpson, M., Buckman, R., Stewart, M. *et al.* (1991). Doctor–patient communication: the Toronto consensus statement. *British Medical Journal*, **303**, 1385–7.

Tattersall, M. and Ellis, P. (1998). Communication is a vital part of care. *British Medical Journal*, **316**, 1891–2.

Towle, A. (1998) Changes in health care and continuing medical education for the 21st Century. *British Medical Journal*, **316**, 301–4.

Tuckett, D., Boulton, M., Olson, C. and Williams A. (1985). *Meetings between Experts. Sharing Ideas and its Importance in Medical Consultations*, Chapter 1. London: Tavistock Publications.

7

Anticipatory care

Robin C. Fraser

By preventing avoidable illness we can
concentrate resources on treating conditions
which cannot yet be prevented (Department
of Health, 1998).

Traditionally, medical education and practice have tended to place a
disproportionate emphasis and value on the ability of doctors to
recognize and manage established disease – to the detriment of seeking
to establish and modify its antecedents. Of course, no one would deny
that diagnostic and treatment skills will always be essential attributes of
clinicians, whether in hospital or in general practice. By themselves,
however, these skills are not enough. For a number of compelling
reasons it is essential that all doctors develop more positive attitudes
towards the undoubted contribution which preventive medicine could
make to improve the health status of the population.

Almost 90 000 people die every year before they reach their 65th
birthday. Of these, nearly 32 000 have cancer and 25 000 die of heart
disease, stroke and related diseases (Department of Health, 1998). Many
of these deaths could be prevented, or at least delayed. Indeed, dramatic
reductions in deaths from ischaemic heart disease and strokes have
occurred in many countries, such as the USA, where appropriate preventive programmes have been vigorously pursued.

Smoking is still the single most important cause of premature death
and disability in the developed world (Bartecchi et al., 1994). For example,
it has been estimated that a cessation of all smoking would result in
reductions in deaths from all cancers and from ischaemic heart disease
of 33% and 25% respectively (Leicestershire Health Authority, 1984).
Furthermore, most instances of bronchitis and emphysema would be
prevented and perinatal mortality reduced. It has also been claimed that
approximately 50% of all strokes could be prevented, mainly through the
early detection and control of high blood pressure (Royal College of
General Practitioners, 1982).

Despite all the evidence, however, medical education and practice still
discriminate in favour of therapeutic medicine, as exemplified by the
following ironic observation made by Gray and Fowler (1983):

Compared with the drama of the coronary care unit, the prevention of myocardial infarction in middle age, by stopping a man in his twenties smoking, is very dull and unglamorous.

Dull and unglamorous it may be, but does it not make sense?

It makes sense because treating preventable illnesses is very expensive. For example, treating heart disease, stroke and related illnesses costs the NHS almost £4 billion every year. A substantial proportion of this sum could well be made available to treat other conditions that cannot yet be prevented, if efforts were concentrated more on preventing avoidable disease. Yet currently only 1% of the NHS budget is spent on health promotion and disease prevention (Speller *et al.*, 1997).

Consequently, clinicians must no longer be satisfied to respond only to the diseases and problems presented to them by patients. Whenever possible, they must be prepared to anticipate the undeclared needs of their patients. Modern doctors need to develop the ability to recognize, *and the conviction to act on*, the opportunities for preventive initiatives available to them in the course of their day-to-day work. To do so effectively and efficiently, they must first understand the concepts and become familiar with the strategies of prevention. General practice provides the optimum setting to observe the scope and practice of anticipatory care.

What is anticipatory care?

The term *anticipatory care* includes all measures that promote good health and prevent or delay the onset of diseases or their complications. Health promotion and disease prevention should be regarded as part of a continuum of activities, the collective aims of which are to:

- Improve the quality of life
- Reduce the burden of premature disability
- Increase life expectancy.

Anticipatory care, therefore, denotes 'the essential union of prevention with care and cure' (Royal College of General Practitioners, 1981). Perhaps the most outstanding example is antenatal care, which is no longer regarded as a different (or lesser) form of care, but as standard clinical practice.

Anticipatory care includes three distinct levels of preventive intervention: primary, secondary and tertiary. This classification reflects the stage in the natural history of a disease where the intervention is made.

- *Primary prevention* aims to prevent altogether the development of a disease process

- *Secondary prevention* involves the early diagnosis of disease – ideally at a presymptomatic stage – followed by prompt and effective treatment
- *Tertiary prevention* is concerned with detecting established, incurable and unreported disease, with a view to minimizing its harmful effects by appropriate treatment and rehabilitation.

Secondary and tertiary forms of prevention should be undertaken only if there is evidence that earlier detection and treatment will produce a more satisfactory outcome than waiting for the patient to present to the doctor. Prime examples are, respectively, cervical cytology and the monitoring of peripheral vascular defects in patients with established diabetes, the most important of which is proliferative retinopathy.

Primary prevention is manifestly more effective than secondary, which in turn is more effective than tertiary. Many of the measures of primary prevention, however, are beyond the control of doctors. For example, one method of primary prevention against the harmful effects of smoking would be a ban on the manufacture and sale of tobacco products. As this is politically rather unlikely, the next step would be to try to persuade people not to start smoking through a range of measures, some involving legislation, others voluntary.

Using the same example, secondary forms of prevention include methods to persuade smokers either to restrict their smoking (e.g. fewer cigarettes, low-tar brands, refrain from inhaling), or to stop smoking altogether early in their smoking careers to forestall the development of chronic bronchitis and other smoking-related diseases.

Finally, tertiary prevention would be directed at patients with established chronic bronchitis, and involve efforts to persuade them to stop smoking in the hope of reducing the rate of deterioration in their lung function. It would also reduce the risk of cancer of the lung, ischaemic heart disease and other smoking-related diseases. This is the form of prevention with which clinicians are already most familiar.

Primary prevention

From the clinician's viewpoint two main techniques are used:

- Health education
- Prophylaxis.

Health education

This approach aims to enlighten people by providing them with information about factors that are known to cause disease, in the hope that they will modify their behaviour by avoiding these risk factors and consequently avoid contracting a particular disease. An example is propaganda against smoking-related diseases.

Prophylaxis
This approach involves a more active medical intervention in an attempt to protect individuals from developing a particular disease; for example, vaccination and immunization procedures.

Secondary prevention

Again, two techniques are used:

- Screening
- Case-finding.

Screening
Screening procedures are systematic attempts to detect undeclared disease in a population of apparently healthy people. Before mounting a screening initiative, certain criteria must first be satisfied (Wilson, 1973):

- The condition sought should be important and recognizable at an early stage in its natural history
- Any screening test used should be practicable and acceptable to patients
- A recognized and effective treatment should exist, and facilities for diagnosis and management should be readily available
- A policy needs to be established on whom to treat
- The cost of screening should be economically balanced against the possible expenditure on medical care as a whole. Once undertaken, screening should be a continuous process.

It must also be remembered that a screening test is not necessarily diagnostic; for example, a random finding of glycosuria is not necessarily indicative of underlying diabetes. The potentially at-risk individual will require a confirmatory test, e.g. a glucose tolerance test.

Case-finding
This is a variant of screening, and is the term used when it is undertaken opportunistically by the doctor responsible for the health care of the individual who is screened. An example of case-finding would be offering to take a middle-aged man's blood pressure when he had attended for treatment for an unrelated condition such as haemorrhoids. This form of prevention is open to all clinicians, and such activities should be concentrated on those particularly at risk. Nevertheless, before undertaking screening or case-finding exercises those responsible are obliged to ensure that benefit and not harm will ensue.

Tertiary prevention

Having ascertained that a patient has an established disease, tertiary preventive measures are concerned with systematic and long-term

monitoring of the patient to prevent or minimize the impact of complications, since it is rarely possible to reverse the disease process. For
patients with hypertension, for example, the principal aim is to avoid
end-organ damage that would otherwise result in stroke, myocardial
infarction or cardiac/renal failure. This requires more than just an
opportunistic approach to individual patients: an organizational framework needs to be established (Hulscher *et al.*, 1997). This should aim to
ensure that all identified hypertensives within practices are regularly
supervized to ensure compliance with treatment, appropriate control of
the level of blood pressure and the avoidance of other risk factors such
as smoking. It is also essential that such a system should be capable of
identifying defaulters so that appropriate action can be taken.

In recognition of the fact that responsibility for the long-term
management of most chronic diseases rests within general practice, many
practices have constructed special registers of patients suffering from
particular conditions such as hypertension, epilepsy, asthma and diabetes. It should be noted, however, that:

> the pre-requisite for high quality control of diabetes is education of
> patients in the nature of their disease, and that this normally requires a
> total of four hours of learning . . . [medical] control and supervision
> probably reach no more than 50% of requirement (Hart, 1981).

Increasingly, special chronic disease management clinics are being
introduced and developed in general practices. and these are frequently
based on evidence-based guidelines and protocols (Grimshaw *et al.*,
1995)

Health promotion

> Health promotion is a multifactorial process operating on individuals
> and communities, through education, prevention and protection measures.
> (Speller *et al.*, 1998).

The notion of health promotion, however, denotes something stronger
than maintaining good health simply by avoiding risk factors for disease.
Health promotion aims to encourage individuals to attain the best possible level of well-being of which they are capable. Consequently, efforts
at health promotion can operate at primary, secondary and tertiary levels
of prevention. For example, at the primary level, increasing numbers of
people are taking active steps to try to prevent heart disease through
regular exercise; for example, there are now some 25 million joggers in
the USA. Even though the achieved reduction in risk may be small, pro-
ponents of this form of health promotion would argue that the resultant
improvement in well-being brought about by regular exercise is worth
the effort.

At the secondary and tertiary levels, health promotion encourages individuals to participate in screening programmes (e.g. regular cervical smears) and to comply with treatment regimes, respectively. The most positive feature of health promotion is that it encourages people to assume responsibility for the maintenance of their own health.

The new role of the clinician in prevention

There are a number of reasons why clinicians – and in particular general practitioners – have a critical part to play nowadays in improving the health status of the population through preventive means. Furthermore, there is mounting pressure on clinicians to practise prevention.

Changes in the pattern of diseases and opportunities for prevention

In the past, advances in the means of prevention of disease and disability owed more to social legislation than to the actions of individual patients or doctors, who had little control over the great infectious diseases. Death rates from infectious diseases were dramatically reduced by, for instance, improved housing, clean water and sewage disposal, long before immunization procedures became available. Thus, decisions taken by Government centrally on behalf of the population could benefit millions of individuals without their direct involvement in the decision-making process.

Today, the situation is very different. The diseases responsible for most disability and deaths (heart disease, strokes, cancer, chronic respiratory diseases) are more chronic and, to a large extent, they are principally determined by the habits and lifestyles of their victims. If what Morris (1982) called the 'rising tide' of premature disability and death is to be turned back, it will require millions of individuals to make their own personal decisions whether or not to adopt a healthier lifestyle and how they will use the health services available to them. As McWhinney (1981) has observed: 'In influencing these decisions, the physician's educational role has assumed a new importance'.

As we shall see later, the most persuasive source of advice is the patient's own general practitioner, although the influence of family and friends will play a part.

The limitations of 'the heroics of salvage'

Many therapeutic and technical advances in medicine have made major and, in some instances, spectacular contributions to the management of established disease – for example, renal dialysis and transplantation. Unfortunately, some of the advances in 'high technology medicine' have tended to benefit comparatively low numbers of patients at an increasing – and sometimes prohibitive – cost. There is a growing realization on the part of government, many doctors and the general public of the law of diminishing returns in relation to the resources allocated to some of the tasks of salvage. It is an uncomfortable fact that, despite all the expensive technical advances, life expectancy for a man aged 30 years has increased by only 5% over the past 25 years or so.

Increasing pressure on doctors to practise prevention

Interest in prevention has been rekindled in and by the government, not least because of the cost explosion in the provision of services to combat diseases. The general public is also becoming increasingly aware of the opportunities for, and benefits of, prevention, and is looking to its medical advisors to provide a lead. Most patients (84%) find discussion of health promotion helpful (Sullivan, 1988), but they do expect the issues raised to be relevant to their presenting problem and wish to reserve the right to accept or reject the advice given (Stott and Pill, 1990).

Pressure on doctors to become more involved in preventive activities has, however, been intensified by a number of recent government initiatives.

In 1991 a strategy of health for England was outlined, which set out a number of specific objectives and targets for improvement in health by the year 2000 (Secretary of State for Health, 1991). This strategy identified *key areas* where improvements in health could be made, and set *targets* within these key areas so that progress could be monitored.

The suggested key areas for action were:

- *Causes of substantial mortality*
  Coronary heart disease
  Stroke
  Cancers
  Accidents
- *Causes of substantial ill health*
  Mental illness
  Diabetes
  Asthma
- *Factors contributing to mortality, ill health, and healthy living*
  Smoking
  Diet and alcohol
  Physical exercise
- *Areas with clear scope for improvement*
  Health of pregnant women, infants and children
  Rehabilitation services for people with a physical disability
  Environmental quality

- *Areas with great potential for harm*
  HIV/AIDS
  Other communicable diseases
  Food safety.

The following are examples of *targets* set for cancer reduction:

- To reduce deaths from breast cancer in women aged 50–64 (the group invited for mammographic screening) by 25% by the year 2000, compared with 1990 values
- To reduce the prevalence of smoking to 22% in men and 21% in women (reductions of 33% and 30% respectively) by the year 2000.

A national breast screening campaign for women aged 50–64 years was introduced and targeted on general practice. The following figures provide some indication of the expected yield (Austoker, 1990):

For 2000 general practice listed patients:
  150 women will be eligible for screening
  7–10 may require further investigations
  2–3 may require a biopsy
  1 may have cancer.

A new NHS Contract for General Practitioners was introduced in 1990 (Health Departments of Great Britain, 1989). Since that time, *all* NHS general practitioners have been required to make available to patients a range of health promotion and preventive activities. These include regular check-ups (for example, annually for the over 75-year-olds) and screening (for example, of blood pressure in newly registered patients). Furthermore, general practitioners received financial incentives to hold a range of health promotion clinics – for example, well-woman clinics, diabetic clinics, coronary heart disease clinics, etc., and for achieving certain target levels for patients receiving immunizations and cervical smears.

In 1998, the new Government set out its preventive health strategy (Department of Health, 1998). The two key aims are:

- To improve the health of the population as a whole by increasing the length of people's lives and the number of years people spend free of illness
- To improve the health of the worst off in society and to narrow the health gap.

This supersedes the previous policy, and sets clear targets for improvement in four priority areas by the year 2010 (baseline 1996). The targets, described in the report as 'tough' and 'challenging', are as follows:

- Heart disease and stroke
  Target: To reduce the death rate from heart disease and stroke and related illnesses aged under 65 years by at least *a further third*
- Accidents
  Target: To reduce accidents (defined here as those that involve a hospital visit or consultation with a family doctor) by at least *a fifth*
- Cancer
  Target: To reduce the death rate from cancer amongst people aged under 65 years by at least *a further fifth*
- Mental health
  Target: To reduce the death rate from suicide and undetermined injury by at least *a further sixth*.

All these factors have influenced, or required, large numbers of general practitioners to initiate a wide range of preventive measures. This, in turn, will influence more of their colleagues to do likewise. It is important, however, that doctors are not pressurized into becoming 'health policemen'.

> Unfortunately . . . offering fees for health checks and screening may place a premium on achieving population coverage rather than encouraging patient-centred plans tailored to the individual's needs over time (Stott and Pill, 1990).

If this happens, there is a danger that:

> the exceptional potential in every primary care consultation can be grossly misused when population coverage becomes more important than patient-centred care (Stott and Pill, 1990).

It is essential, therefore, for doctors to retain a sense of balance in undertaking and pursuing potential preventive initiatives. It is required behaviour for doctors to provide patients with appropriate information and advice to enable them to choose paths of action for themselves (see Chapter 8). It would be entirely unacceptable, however, for doctors to attempt to coerce patients to adhere to arbitrary norms of approved behaviour as handed down by governments.

General practice: the optimum setting for anticipatory care

The general practitioner has been described as 'the key to preventive medicine' (Gray and Fowler, 1983). Because of the primary, personal, comprehensive and continuing nature of care in general practice (see Chapter 1), it possesses characteristics which make it an ideal setting for delivering effective anticipatory care at primary, secondary and tertiary levels. These include the following.

Frequent contacts between doctor and patient over many years

- The average number of doctor–patient contacts each year is 3–4
- Approximately 10% of the contacts take place in the patient's own home
- About 80% of patients consult their general practitioner at least once a year
- More than 90% of patients consult their general practitioner at least once every 5 years
- There are more than one million face-to-face consultations between general practitioners and their patients every day in the UK
- 78% of patients remain with the same doctor for 5 years or more
- 42% of patients remain with the same doctor for 20 years or more
- A significant minority of patients will remain patients of the same practice all their lives.

Every consultation provides an opportunity for effective preventive action, and home visits provide even greater opportunities. Repeated contacts with the same patients and other members of the family provide repeated opportunities for reinforcement.

Responsibility for a defined population

Over 98% of the British population are individually registered with a personal general practitioner within the National Health Service. It is possible, therefore, to construct an age–sex register, which is an index of the total practice population classified by age and sex. The age–sex register can be used to identify at-risk groups among a general practitioner's patients – *whether they consult or not.*

It is possible also to construct at-risk registers. Suitable for inclusion in such registers would be patients with conditions in need of long-term supervision, e.g. diabetics, victims of child abuse, etc.

The general practitioner with an age–sex register is, therefore, the only clinician who has the capability to provide anticipatory care for a population of patients, and who can gain access to patients who might not attend on their own initiative but who may be particularly at risk. Over 80% of practices have age–sex registers.

The contribution of the primary care team

In discharging their preventive responsibilities to their practice population, general practitioners are greatly supported and assisted by the other members of the primary care team (see Chapter 1).

Every member of the team has a particular set of functions, although the health visitor is the only one with the sole task of providing preventive services, mainly for under-5s and the elderly. All the other members of the team combine preventive and therapeutic roles to differing extents, although many practice-employed nurses spend a considerable proportion of their time in chronic disease management (tertiary prevention).

The power of the doctor–patient relationship

Because of the nature of general practice, very close relationships tend to develop between general practitioners and their patients (see Chapter 5). As an influence on compliance, the doctor–patient relationship is paramount (Pendleton et al., 1983). The better the relationship, the more likely the patient is to comply with advice from the doctor regarding both prevention and treatment.

Indeed, it has been shown that:

> Of all the many and varied sources of health information available to the adult population, it is the general practitioner who is most trusted and whose advice has most impact (McCron and Budd, 1979; unpublished).

Nevertheless, it needs to be firmly stressed that the powers of persuasion of a general practitioner are not limitless. If a patient has made a decision and does not wish to give up smoking, no amount of persuasion or cajoling from a doctor will succeed in altering these circumstances (Butler et al., 1998).

Observing prevention in action

As the range of possible preventive activities is so wide, no single practice can undertake or demonstrate all of them. Consequently choices have to be made, and these will reflect both the interests and motivation of the doctors as well as the needs of their patients. The Royal College of General Practitioners (1981) has recommended a long list of opportunities for prevention, the most worthwhile of which are: family planning, antenatal care, immunization, fostering the bonds between mother and child, discouragement of smoking, detection and management of raised blood pressure, and helping the bereaved. To what extent are these activities carried out in your teaching practice? What are the particular preventive interests in your teaching practice? Why have they been chosen?

During your practice attachment you should have ample opportunity to set yourself some tasks and seek answers to further questions, such as the following:

- To what extent is anticipatory care carried out:
  a. on an opportunistic basis within the consultation?
  b. on a systematic basis for the practice population?
- How is an age–sex register used for prevention?
- How is immunization/cervical cytology carried out?
- Attend an antenatal clinic: what problems affecting the mother and/or fetus should be detected by antenatal care?
- Interview and observe the health visitor at work. How do health visitors see their role?
- Observe and record how the general practitioner deals with a woman on an oral contraceptive
- How would you advise anxious parents enquiring about whooping cough immunization for their child?

Key points

- Anticipatory care consists of health promotion and disease prevention.
- It denotes the integration of prevention, care and cure.
- The answer to our present killing and disabling diseases is prevention, not cure.
- The setting of general practice provides the best opportunity for observing preventive opportunities and implementing preventive actions.
- Clinicians, particularly general practitioners, must discharge their new role in prevention more actively.
- Opportunistic anticipatory care initiatives must target receptive individuals and avoid preaching.

References

Austoker, J. (1990). Breast screening and the primary care team. *British Medical Journal*, 300, 1631.

Bartecchi, C. E., Mackenzie, T. D. and Schrier, R. W. (1994). The human costs of tobacco use (Part 1). *New England Journal of Medicine*, 330, 907–12.

Butler, C. C., Pill, R. and Stott, N. H. C. (1998). Qualitative study of patients' perceptions of doctors' advice to quit smoking: implications for opportunistic health promotion. *British Medical Journal*, 316, 1878–81.

Department of Health (1998). *Our Healthier Nation: A Contract for Health*. London: HMSO (CM3852).

Gray, J. A. M. and Fowler, G. H. (1983). *Preventive Medicine in General Practice*, p. 286. Oxford: Oxford University Press.

Grimshaw, J., Freemantle, N., Wallace, S. *et al.* (1995). Developing and implementing clinical practice guidelines. *Quality in Health Care*, 4, 55–64.

Hart, J. T. (1981). A new kind of doctor. *Journal of the Royal Society of Medicine*, 74, 871.

Health Departments of Great Britain (1989). *General Practice in the National Health Service: The 1990 Contract*. London: HMSO.

Hulscher, M. E. J. L., Drenth, B. B., Mokkink, H. G. A. *et al.*, (1997). Barriers to preventive care in general practice: the role of organizational and attitudinal factors. *British Journal of General Practice*, **47**, 711–14.

Leicestershire Health Authority (1984). *Health Promotion, Health Education and Disease Prevention*. Addendum to the Strategic Intentions Document 1984–1994.

McWhinney, I. R. (1981). *An Introduction to Family Medicine*, p. 216. Oxford: Oxford University Press.

Morris, J. N. (1982). Prospects for health promotion. In *Progress in Health Promotion: United Kingdom and Abroad*. Leicester: Faculty of Community Medicine, Leicester University.

Pendleton, D., Tate, P., Havelock, P. and Schofield, T. (1983). *The Consultation: An Approach to Learning and Teaching*. Oxford: Oxford University Press.

Royal College of General Practitioners (1981). *Health and Prevention in Primary Care*. Report from General Practice no. 18 (plus three further reports relating to children, arterial disease and psychiatric disorders respectively). London: RCGP.

Royal College of General Practitioners (1982). *The Prevention of Arterial Disease*. Report from General Practice no. 19, London: RCGP.

Secretary of State for Health (1991). *The Health of the Nation*. CM1523. London: HMSO.

Speller, V., Learmonth, A. and Harrison, D. (1997). The search for evidence of effective health promotion. *British Medical Journal*, **315**, 361–3.

Stott, N. C. H. and Pill, R. M. (1990). Advise yes, dictate no! Patients' views on health promotion in the consultation. *Family Practice*, **7**, 125.

Sullivan, D. (1988). Opportunistic health promotion: do patients like it? *Journal of the Royal College of General Practitioners*, **38**, 24.

Wilson, J. M. G. (1973). Screening for disease. In *A Companion to Medical Studies*. (R. Passmore and J. S. Robson, eds.), Vol 3/2, Chapter 76. Oxford: Blackwell Scientific.

8

A systematic approach in the consultation to lifestyle modification: helping patients to stop smoking

Robin C. Fraser and Timothy J. Coleman

... Patients resent doctors dictating to them
about lifestyle change ... action oriented
advice for those who are not ready to change
is at best unhelpful and could even entrench
unhealthy behaviour (Butler *et al.*, 1998).

The previous chapter outlined the fundamental concepts and principles of health promotion and disease prevention, and this chapter aims to illustrate how they can be applied to the modification of patient lifestyles in everyday clinical practice. This is because many of the present killing and disabling diseases are directly linked to unhealthy lifestyles related to, for example, diet, physical activity, sexual behaviour, smoking, alcohol and drugs. Consequently, the clinician's role is increasingly to assist people to make appropriate changes in their lifestyle which will enable them to live healthier – and longer – lives. It is our intention to consider one lifestyle modification topic in detail, i.e. stopping smoking, as it can be adopted by clinicians as a model when attempting to encourage patients to make other health-related lifestyle changes.

The model will exemplify the following aspects of any health-related lifestyle modification process:

- Patients differ widely in their motivation to change
- Attention should be particularly focused on motivated patients
- Patients should be involved in setting their own targets for behaviour change
- Advice from the doctor should be based on sound evidence rather than unsubstantiated opinion
- The provision of continuing support through review of progress and reinforcement is essential to successful lifestyle modification
- The attitude and style of the doctor has a direct bearing on success or failure in influencing patients to make lifestyle changes.

We have selected smoking cessation as the model topic for two main reasons. First, stopping smoking is the single most important behavioural change which clinicians can encourage patients to make, since smoking is the major risk factor for premature death and disability, which is capable of modification. Second, it has been shown that general practice is an effective context for influencing patients to stop smoking through opportunistic intervention as patients consult.

There is a compelling catalogue of evidence of the harmful effects of smoking:

> . . . Of every 1000 young smokers, one will be murdered, six will be killed in a road accident and 250 will die before their time because they smoke (Department of Health, 1998).

Following 40 years of observation of 35 000 British doctors, it has been concluded that of those who die in middle age because of smoking, the average loss of life expectancy is 20–25 years (Doll and Peto, 1994). Twenty-six per cent of smokers die from lung cancer and 25% from heart disease, and yet 29% of men and 27% of women over the age of 16 years in the UK still smoke (Office of Population Censuses and Surveys, 1994).

> Clearly, smoking tobacco remains an enormous public health problem which requires an appropriate response from all clinicians when encountering patients who smoke (Coleman and Lakhani, 1998).

General practitioners can make a particular contribution to the provision of effective anti-smoking advice to patients, as it has been demonstrated that two out of every 50 smokers advised to stop by their general practitioners will succeed in doing so (Ashenden *et al.*, 1997). Furthermore, reinforcement with consistent anti-smoking messages from other primary health care team (PHCT) members can be similarly effective.

Prevention in the consultation: some important factors

The essential tasks of the clinician are to recognize appropriate preventive opportunities, to communicate information to patients in a readily understandable fashion, and to provide ongoing support in the hope that patients will be persuaded to change their behaviour towards a healthier lifestyle. The particular consultation competences that need to be acquired are outlined in Chapter 2 (anticipatory care consultation category). The extent to which the giving of preventive advice – particularly at secondary and tertiary levels of prevention – will be followed by an appropriate change of behaviour depends on the health beliefs of the individual and the source of the advice. Compliance with advice tends to have a positive association with the following factors (Gray and Fowler, 1983):

- The seriousness of the specific disease
- The perceived susceptibility of an individual patient to the specific disease
- The perceived susceptibility of the patient to disease in general
- The efficacy of advice/therapy.

There is also growing evidence that patients require their doctors to show a caring, individualized approach when raising preventive issues in the consultation (Butler *et al.*, 1998). Patients prefer their doctor to:

- Take account of their degree of receptiveness to change in their lifestyle
- Discuss preventive issues in a respectful tone
- Avoid preaching.

Furthermore, research studies have identified four key elements of clinical care that contribute towards successful anti-smoking interventions (Fiore *et al.*, 1996). It is essential that clinicians:

- Regularly ascertain and document information on patients' smoking habits
- Determine smokers' motivation to stop
- Are familiar with simple and effective anti-smoking interventions
- Are prepared to provide reinforcement of interventions through continuing follow-up, as this increases the success rate of smokers who try to stop.

Helping patients to stop smoking: a systematic approach

Figure 8.1 outlines a practical and systematic approach to helping patients to stop smoking. Smokers must first of all be identified, their motivation to stop assessed, and an evidence-based action plan negotiated and agreed with those motivated to stop: this should include appropriate follow-up. These steps will now be considered in greater detail.

Identifying patients who smoke

It is helpful and sensible to establish at the outset whether or not a consulting patient smokes. As part of your review of a patient's record

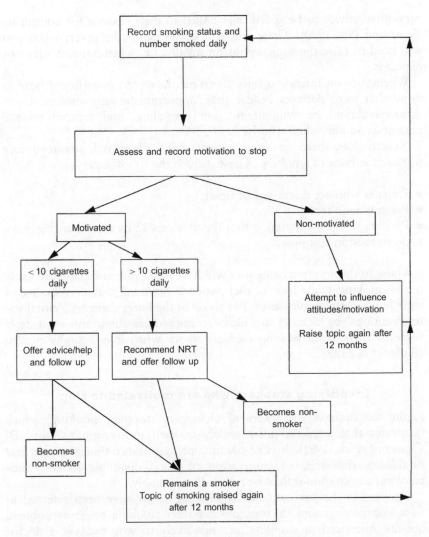

Figure 8.1 Helping patients to stop smoking: a systematic approach (adapted from Coleman and Lakhani, 1998)

prior to every consultation (see Chapter 3), you should ascertain whether smoking status has been recorded. If the notes contain no such information, clinical cues can be used to identify smokers; for example, smell of tobacco from clothes and/or breath, or nicotine-stained fingers and/or teeth.

In the absence of specific information or cues, you will have to ask patients directly (but sensitively) about their smoking habits. Many patients presenting with smoking-related problems, including pregnancy, will expect the issue of smoking to be raised, and many patients prefer preventive advice to be specifically linked to their reasons for consulting (Stott and Pill, 1990). There will still be occasions, however, when you will need to raise the topic opportunistically, i.e. when patients may not expect it.

Whenever you intend to raise the topic, however, you should bear in mind that most patients believe that 'opportunistic anti-smoking interventions should be sympathetic, not preaching, and centred on the patient as an individual' (Butler *et al*., 1998).

Nevertheless, there are some patients with whom it is *inappropriate* to raise the issue of smoking. These include the following:

• Patients who are distressed or upset
• Patients with terminal illness
• Patients who have stated within the previous 12 months that they have no interest in stopping.

Those in the first two categories will have other priorities, and are likely to see smoking as the least of their worries. Smoking may even be one of their few remaining pleasures. For those in the latter category, 'ritualistic interventions' by doctors are likely to antagonize them and even deter some of them from seeking medical advice when it is actually needed (Butler *et al*., 1998).

Identifying smokers who are motivated to stop

Figure 8.2 outlines the stages of change in stopping smoking, which illustrates that smokers differ widely in their motivation to stop (Di Clemente *et al*., 1991). It is of paramount importance that a doctor *first* establishes the stage of motivation of the individual smoker; anti-smoking advice should then be tailored accordingly.

Smokers in the *pre-contemplation stage* (who have been referred to as a 'contrary' group) do not consider their smoking to be a problem, are not interested in stopping, are not likely to stop because a doctor tells them to, are already saturated with anti-smoking information and may even smoke more in response to being told to stop (Butler *et al*., 1998). There is no point, therefore, in trying to urge a pre-contemplator to set a date for stopping smoking, as these smokers lack the motivation to take the necessary action. Furthermore, it also appears that the patients of today are fully aware of the dangers of smoking and feel that it is up to them as individuals to decide whether or not to try to stop (Butler *et al*., 1998). Again, there is no point in trying to harangue such patients with horrific tales of the harmful long-term effects of smoking.

In the consultation, therefore, first establish whether a smoker wishes to stop. If the answer is 'no' do not pursue the issue (beyond recording the fact in the patient's notes), but consider raising it again after an

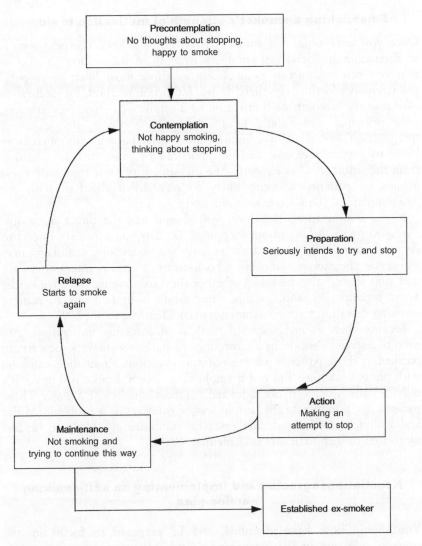

Figure 8.2 Stages of change in stopping smoking (adapted from Di Clemente *et al.*, 1991)

interval of 12 months (see Figure 8.1) as the patient's views *may* have changed. In the meantime, you may wish to attempt the difficult task of trying to encourage the non-motivated to develop negative attitudes towards their smoking by focusing on the short-term harm caused by it when such patients consult with cough, sore throat, etc.

A particular group that should be targeted is that of smokers who become pregnant, as this is likely to make them more motivated to stop (Dolan-Mullen *et al.*, 1994).

Establishing a smoker's strength of motivation to stop

Once you have separated smokers from non-smokers, the next step is to determine an individual smoker's strength of motivation to stop so that you can concentrate your efforts on those most likely to respond positively. Unfortunately there is no foolproof method for accurately assessing the strength of motivation of a smoker to stop. Nevertheless, your principal aim should be to determine those at the stages of 'preparation' or 'action' (see Figure 8.2), as these patients are much more likely to expect, welcome and be influenced by preventive intervention from their doctor. Consequently, the investment of your time with these groups of patients is more likely to pay dividends than with the 'contemplators' (Di Clemente *et al.*, 1991).

In the consultation, therefore, you should ask the direct questions: 'Are you just *thinking* about stopping?' or 'Do you *seriously* intend to try and stop?'. By their answers to these questions, smokers may categorize themselves. Smokers who indicate a serious intention to try and stop should also be asked whether they are making (or have made) active attempts to stop, as this latter group is more likely to achieve smoking cessation than contemplators (Di Clemente *et al.*, 1991).

Because there is no foolproof method of assessing motivation, you need to exercise caution in interpreting the patient's answers. Beware, in particular, those patients who respond to questions about their smoking with phrases such as 'I'm not a smoker . . . I only smoke roll-ups', 'It's only a habit . . . I'm not addicted', 'I only smoke 30 a day'. These patients are minimizing the seriousness of smoking as a problem (Miller and Rollnick, 1991), and smokers who minimize are likely to be less motivated to stop than others (Coleman, 1998).

Negotiating, agreeing and implementing an anti-smoking action plan

You should now have identified, and be prepared to focus on, the smokers who are in the 'preparation' and 'action' stages of stopping. These patients will probably be aware of the harm that smoking is doing, and can do, to them. However, if you feel (or the patient indicates) that more information is needed about the harmful effects of smoking, then be prepared to provide it.

You should then negotiate and agree an action plan with the patient. This should be based on supporting evidence for the effectiveness of any suggested intervention, since it would be unethical for a doctor to advise patients to change their lifestyle if based on personal opinion only. Aim to negotiate achievable targets for stopping with individual smokers, according to their own circumstances, as those who feel in control of their efforts to stop are more likely to be successful. *Encouraging smokers to attain targets which they have helped to select will be more* effective than *telling* them what to do. Where smokers are happy to set a date for stopping, you should agree a particular date. However, if a patient wishes to take more modest action (for example, reducing daily consumption, refraining from inhaling or switching to lower tar brands), you should support them in this with a view to stopping completely at a later, but as yet unspecified, date. Whatever action plan is agreed with the patient, it is useful to reinforce it with the provision of anti-smoking leaflets, as they potentiate the effects of any verbal advice given (Russell *et al.*, 1979).

You should inform patients that they may experience physical withdrawal symptoms such as irritability and/or craving for a cigarette (Lennox, 1992), but reassure them that these will usually abate in approximately 2 weeks (Mendelsohn and Richmond, 1992). Further encourage your patients by explaining to them that most smokers who manage to stop for 4 months will not restart (Marlatt *et al.*, 1988).

Many patients worry about weight gain as a consequence of giving up smoking. You should acknowledge that this is perhaps likely, but not inevitable, and explain that the average weight gain is less than 5 kg (Fiore *et al.*, 1996). You should advise them, however, not to attempt strict dieting during a stop-smoking attempt, as this might put them under too much pressure. Any attempt at losing weight should be postponed until the individual patient is confident of not restarting smoking.

An 8-week course of nicotine replacement therapy (NRT) should be recommended to motivated patients who consume more than 10 cigarettes daily, as it has been shown that this will double success rates (Silagy *et al.*, 1997). In this regard, nicotine patches and nicotine chewing gum are equally effective. You should advise those who smoke 10 or less cigarettes daily that they will not benefit from NRT, the only exception being patients who are particularly concerned about the prospect of weight gain (see above). There is strong evidence that NRT helps to postpone weight gain in such patients (Fiore *et al.*, 1996) and, accordingly, they can be advised to use it until, as an ex-smoker, they feel able to follow a weight control strategy.

You should *always* offer follow-up, either with a doctor or another member of the PHCT, to all patients who have agreed actively to try and stop smoking. This is because the greater contact smokers have with those advising them against smoking, the more likely they are to stop (Ashenden *et al.*, 1997). Follow-up allows you to monitor the patient's progress, re-inforce the 'stop-smoking message', and agree any appropriate modifications to the action plan. Continuing support is also essential for the successful use of NRT.

Finally, you should bear in mind that it is unusual for smokers to stop completely at their first attempt (Marsh and Matheson, 1983). If relapse occurs, you should be tolerant and indicate that you are prepared to provide continuing support if the patient is still motivated to make a further attempt to stop.

Key points

- Smoking is the major risk factor for premature death and disability in the developed world.
- Consequently, stopping smoking is the single most important behavioural change doctors can encourage and assist patients to make.
- Doctors must adopt a systematic approach to identifying and assisting those smokers who are most motivated to stop.
- The suggested approach for identifying smokers, categorizing those most motivated to stop and negotiating, agreeing and implementing an action plan (to include continuing support and reinforcement) can be used as a model for other lifestyle behaviour modification topics.
- Lifestyle modification advice from doctors should be based on sound evidence of effectiveness rather than unsubstantiated personal opinion.
- Patients expect doctors to adopt a caring, individualized approach when raising preventive issues – they resent doctors dictating to them about lifestyle change.

References

Ashenden, R., Silagy, C. and Weller, D. (1997). A systematic review of the effectiveness of promoting lifestyle change in general practice. *Family Practice*, **14**, 160–76.

Butler, C. C., Pill, R. and Stott, N. H. C. (1998). Qualitative study of patients' perceptions of doctors' advice to quit smoking: implications for opportunistic health promotion. *British Medical Journal*, **316**, 1878–81.

Coleman, T. and Lakhani, M. K. (1998). Improving health promotion activity: a protocol for an audit of helping patients to stop smoking. In *Evidence-Based Audit in General Practice: From Principles to Practice* (R. C. Fraser, M. K. Lakhani and R. H. Baker, eds.), pp. 73–82. Oxford: Butterworth-Heinemann.

Coleman, T. (1998). Anti-smoking advice in general practice consultations: a description of factors influencing provision of advice and the development of a method for describing smokers' responses. MD thesis, University of Leicester.

Department of Health (1998). *Our Healthier Nation: A Contract for Health*. London: HMSO (CM3852).

Di Clemente, C. C., Prochaska, J. O., Fairhurst, S. K. *et al.* (1991). The process of smoking cessation: an analysis of precontemplation, contemplation, and preparation stages of change. *Journal of Consulting and Clinical Psychology*, **59**, 295–304.

Dolan-Mullen, P., Ramirez, G. and Groff, J. Y. (1994). A meta-analysis of randomized trials of prenatal smoking cessation interventions. *American Journal of Obstetrics and Gynaecology*, **171**(5), 1328–34.

Doll, R. and Peto, R. (1994). Mortality in relation to smoking: 40 years of observation in male British doctors. *British Medical Journal*, **309**, 901–11.

Fiore, M. C., Bailey, W. C., Cohen, S. J. *et al.* (1996). *Smoking Cessation. Clinical Practice Guideline No. 18*. Rockville, MD: US Department of Health and Human Services, Public Health Service/Agency for Health Care Policy and Research (AHCPR) Publication No. 96-0692).

Gray, J. A. M. and Fowler, G. H. (1983). *Preventive Medicine in General Practice*, p. 268. Oxford: Oxford University Press.

Lennox, A. S. (1992). Determinants of outcome in smoking cessation. *British Journal of General Practice*, **42**, 247–52.

Marlatt, G. A., Curry, S. and Gordon, R. (1988). A longitudinal analysis of unaided smoking cessation. *Journal of Consulting and Clinical Psychology*, **56**, 715–20.

Marsh, A. and Matheson, J. (1983). *Smoking Attitudes and Behaviour*, pp. 118–126. London: HMSO.

Mendelsohn, C. P. and Richmond, R. (1992). GPs can help patients to stop smoking. *Medical Journal of Australia*, **157**(7), 463–7.

Miller, W. R. and Rollnick, S. (1991) *Motivational Interviewing: Preparing People to Change Addictive Behaviour*. New York: Guildford Press.

Office of Population Censuses and Surveys (1994). *General Household Survey 1992 (Series GHS, No.23, GB, Age 16+)*. London: HMSO.

Russell, M. A. H., Wilson, C., Taylor, C. and Baker, C. B. (1979). Effect of GPs' advice against smoking. *British Medical Journal*, **2**, 231–5.

Silagy, D., Mant, D., Fowler, G. and Lancaster, T. (1997). The effect of nicotine replacement therapy on smoking cessation. In: *Tobacco Addiction Module of The Cochrane Database of Systematic Reviews* (T. Lancaster, C. Silagy and D. Fullerton), updated 03 March 1998 (updated quarterly). Available in The Cochrane Library (database on disk and CD ROM). The Cochrane Collaboration; Issue 2. Oxford: Update Software.

Stott, N. C. H. and Pill, R. M. (1990). Advise yes, dictate no! Patients' views on health promotion in the consultation. *Family Practice*, **7**, 125.

9
Ethics in practice

Robert K. McKinley and Pauline A. McAvoy

> . . . all clinical or professional decisions have
> a moral aspect to them, for morality, like
> attitudes, is all pervasive (Downie and
> Calman, 1994).

Ethics is the study of rational and moral processes for determining the best course of action in the face of conflicting choices. It is therefore concerned with human character and rules of behaviour. *Medical ethics* is that part of ethics specifically concerned with the professional standards and behaviour of doctors.

Medical ethics is not a modern discipline. The Hippocratic oath, written in the 4th Century BC (Johnson, 1990a), is an early attempt to formalize the responsibilities and duties of physicians. It describes their responsibilities to their patients, their teachers and their pupils. These have been revised and amplified by later statements on ethics, for example the Geneva declaration of 1968 (Johnson, 1990b) and the Helsinki declaration of 1975 (Johnson, 1990c). However, increasing opportunities and temptations for doctors to 'play God' have arisen with, for example, *in-vitro* fertilization and 'extraordinary' life-sustaining technology, and these have forced doctors to examine their professional values and actions as never before. Nevertheless, it is important to stress that ethics are not just the concern of those working at the boundaries of medicine. Increasingly, day-to-day decisions raise ethical dilemmas that affect *all* doctors, whether researcher, hospital doctor, general practitioner or administrative physician. Consequently, it is essential to equip all doctors with the necessary skills to enable them to recognize the dilemmas which they will eventually encounter in their work so that they can analyse them, arrive at sound conclusions and take appropriate actions.

Various approaches could be taken to introduce medical ethics to undergraduates. Our preferred approach is to assist the reader to develop an understanding of fundamental and generic ethical issues, which can then be applied to particular situations using a 'problem-solving' framework. This chapter will therefore provide an introduction to basic ethical principles and illustrate how these can be applied in clinical practice.

Fundamental ethical principles in health care

There are three fundamental principles which are of over-riding importance in medical ethics (Thompson, 1987);

- Justice (or equity)
- Respect for persons
- Beneficence.

Justice (or equity)

This principle demands that no-one is discriminated against on the grounds of age, sex, race or social or economic standing. It ensures that the weak or vulnerable (for whatever reason and in whatever situation) will not be disadvantaged. Justice in this context is concerned with the fair distribution of resources of any kind, whether they be material resources, expertise or time. It does not involve either punishment or reward. Justice can be concerned with the individual or with groups; for example, the provision of care to a vagrant or health care of the underprivileged.

Respect for persons

Respect for persons has four inter-related components.

- *Respect for autonomy* means that people must be allowed to control their destiny. Even if a person is unconscious or has intellectual impairment and is not capable of exerting such control, autonomy is reduced but not absent. In these situations, care must be taken to ensure that actions taken on patients' behalf do not offend their known desires or wishes.
- *Informed consent* means that individuals must have the opportunity to make a real decision about any course of action they are going to undertake, or which will be undertaken on their behalf. Furthermore, all essential information to help patients make any decision must be provided. If any necessary information is withheld, consent cannot be informed. The definition of 'necessary information' in medicine is difficult. In some societies there is a duty to provide patients with all the information about the effects and side-effects of a treatment and its alternatives. In the United Kingdom, the duty to provide inform-ation has been limited to 'what a responsible body of medical men' (Gillon, 1986a) would provide, unless there is a significant risk associated with the treatment, when patients should be informed of that risk. The requirement to obtain informed consent is also part of respect for autonomy.
- *Truth-telling* is related intimately to autonomy and to informed consent. People who have been lied to lose control of part of their life

because of the lack of relevant information. It follows, therefore, that permission for the course of action being discussed will not be valid.

- *Respect for confidentiality* means that individuals who have given information to a doctor expecting that it will be kept private or in confidence continue to 'own' that information. Consequently, the doctor is not permitted to divulge this information without the patient's informed consent, usually in writing.

Beneficence

This is assumed to encompass both doing good for the patient (beneficence), and not harming the patient (non-maleficence). Although these notions are complementary they can also be contradictory, but cannot be regarded as opposites (see below). Thompson (1987) has widened the concept of beneficence to encompass the duty to inform and educate. Education will enhance patients' ability to self-care so that the beneficent act can continue.

In some situations these principles may conflict with each other, and a balance has to be struck between them. For example, conflict between beneficence and non-maleficence arises when considering the benefits and side-effects of treatment. Beneficence demands that the doctor does good, but non-maleficence demands that no harm is done. What happens if a proposed treatment has a possible severe adverse reaction? Does the need to do good over-ride the demand to do no harm? The balance of these conflicts will depend on the patient, the severity of the illness and the likely frequency of occurrence of the adverse reaction. The oral contraceptive pill is an extremely safe medication but, because it is usually taken by healthy females, a very low level of potential adverse reactions is required before the conflict between benefit and harm is resolved. When considering a patient with temporal arteritis, however, the considerable risks associated with high-dose steroid treatment in an elderly patient (hypertension, impaired glucose tolerance, peptic ulceration) are acceptable because treatment will prevent major permanent disability (blindness) and cure a potentially serious illness.

Ethics and context

In clinical medicine, ethical problems do not exist in isolation; both the doctor and the patient need to be considered.

The patient

The patient, rather than the ethics of the situation, should be the major consideration. Each situation is unique, and there can be no general solution for all situations. This has been hinted at in the discussion of beneficence and non-maleficence above. In the case of immunization, a child with a strong family history of asthma who lives in poor and overcrowded housing is at higher risk of contracting and suffering long-term harm from pertussis than a child from a professional family with good housing and no family history of respiratory disease. Therefore, the balance of the debate on whether immunization should be carried out will be different in each case. This must be borne in mind by the doctor in all situations where ethical dilemmas arise.

The doctor

Although patients and their circumstances are the most important considerations in the ethical analysis of a problem, doctors must not be ignored. Like patients, doctors each have a unique set of values and experiences determined by their social and cultural backgrounds. These affect the negotiated solution chosen, which must take into account the doctor's personal values. Conversely, doctors must be aware of these values and how they affect their decision-making, since doctors have a duty to ensure that patients will not be disadvantaged by them.

Solving ethical problems

There is not necessarily a 'correct' analysis and decision to apply to a problem. Indeed, different interpretations can illuminate the dilemma. For example, when considering immunization of a child, the principle of justice would encourage the immunization of the child because it is protective and an efficient and equitable use of resources. The application of the principle of non-maleficence may insist that the risks of vaccine damage are unacceptable and the child should not be immunized. Beneficence would require us to administer the vaccine to decrease the risk of morbidity and possible mortality of the child contracting the infection. How then does a doctor choose an appropriate analysis and action? Brody (1981) proposed a method of ethical reasoning in which decisions between potential actions depend on the consequences of the potential actions. The first step is to make sure that a dilemma exists. This requires that:

- A *real* choice exists between possible courses of action; if not a dilemma cannot exist.
- The person involved must place a significantly different value upon the potential actions or consequences. If the differences do not matter either to those involved or to society, then it is not an ethical dilemma but a matter of personal preference.

The next step is to describe alternative courses of action. To do this, the following issues should be considered:

- What is to be done? (What?)
- Who is to do it? (Who?)
- The conditions under which the statement is applicable (When?).

A description of a course of action might read: 'The doctor (who) ought to provide termination in pregnancy (what) for any woman who requests it (when)'. An alternative course of action could be 'The doctor (who) ought to provide termination in pregnancy (what) only when the mother's life is at serious risk because of the pregnancy (when)'. We do not imply, however, that there are only two alternatives for each dilemma; seldom is the practice of medicine so straightforward!

The practitioner's preferred course of action should be evaluated by examining its consequences on whoever might be affected by it and the consequences set against the doctor's personal and professional values. If there are no disagreements, the action is ethically acceptable. If there are, however, the proposed course of action must either be modified or rejected and an alternative examined using the same criteria. The three fundamental ethical principles (equity, autonomy and beneficence) should be used as guidelines to ensure that all major areas of potential ethical conflict are considered. This process of selection, examination, modification or reselection and re-examination is continued until a satisfactory course of action is produced.

This process of testing, modification or rejection and selection is analogous to the hypothetico-deductive method of clinical problem solving described in Chapter 3.

Ethical problems raised and discussed with students are usually based on cases which have made headline news; for example, the 'Arthur case' (Gillon 1986b), the 'Gillick case' (Johnson 1990d), 'Child B' (Price 1996), *in-vitro* fertilization or surrogate motherhood. However, the day-to-day work of a general practitioner or hospital clinician is filled with ethical problems that require recognition and solution.

Example 1

Mrs Smith, a mother of four children, is opportunistically offered diphtheria, pertussis and tetanus (DPT) and polio immunization for John, her youngest child, after failing to attend the immunization clinic on two occasions. Mr Smith is unemployed and has asthma. Both parents smoke. Ryan, the eldest child (aged 6 years), has asthma and eczema, and both John and Mary (the second child) have eczema. Mrs Smith refuses pertussis immunization on the grounds that her sister had a febrile convulsion and Ryan had a fever after his DPT immunization.

There are several possible theoretical courses of action;

- The doctor could immunize all children for diphtheria, pertussis, tetanus and polio irrespective of the parents' wishes.

- The doctor could respect the parents' wishes with regard to immunizations.
- The doctor could attempt to educate the parents appropriately, and then respect the fully informed wishes of the parents with regard to immunization.

Immunization is an efficient and equitable use of resources, can prevent morbidity and mortality for the child and others (beneficence) at the risk of some minor side-effects and rare major side-effects (maleficence). The principle of respect for persons is complicated because John is incapable of giving consent and his parents therefore have to give permission for his treatment. However, the combination of an aunt who had a febrile convulsion and a sibling who had a fever after immunization is not a contraindication to DPT administration. Mrs Smith is therefore basing her refusal to give consent on a false premise, but it is important to realize that this does not make her refusal invalid.

With regard to option (1), the immediate consequence of immunizing John against Mrs Smith's express wishes is that the doctor would have committed an assault on John and this is obviously unacceptable to the child, parent, society and the doctor. Thus, option (1) is a theoretical one only, since no doctor would seriously consider immunizing children against their parents' wishes.

The consequences of accepting Mrs Smith's refusal (option 2) are that John, who is at relatively high risk of contracting pertussis and suffering long-term effects, will not be given all available protection against an infection which could harm him; on the other hand, the risk of a rare serious reaction will be avoided. These consequences may be acceptable to some doctors but not all. Alternatively, if the doctor attempts to educate Mrs Smith about the true contraindications to immunization and its relative risks and benefits and succeeds in obtaining her informed consent, the benefits of immunization will be achieved. The information given to Mrs Smith must be correct and in context.

Example 2

A 29-year-old, fit, healthy, non-smoking, married accountant using the oral contraceptive pill requests a cervical smear. She has no history of other risk factors for cervical cancer. Her last smear was normal 2 years previously. She has read, however, that women on the 'pill' have a higher risk of developing cervical cancer. She has also heard that younger women can develop a rapidly progressive form of cervical cancer, which could only be detected early if screening were carried out more frequently than every 3 years.

Try to formulate alternative ways of responding to this problem, making appropriate reference to the ethical principles involved (see the appendix to this chapter regarding potential courses of action).

Example 3

John Smyth, a 38-year-old computer salesman, attends his general practitioner complaining of a few days' discomfort passing urine since returning from a conference abroad. Both he and his wife, Sally, are patients of the practice. They have been married for 5 years and have been investigated for infertility, for which no cause has been found. Investigation establishes the presence of a chlamydia infection. At review, the doctor suggests that Sally should be told because, if she is not properly diagnosed, treated and followed up, she could suffer long-term harm. John insists that he does not want his wife to know because their marriage is in difficulty, and that this could be the last straw.

Again, try to formulate alternative ways of responding to this problem, making appropriate reference to the ethical principles involved (see the appendix to this chapter regarding potential courses of action).

Conclusion

All doctors must be aware of the increasing potential for ethical conflict in their work. They must be aware that their analysis of a dilemma will depend on personal weightings of factors which bear on the situation. This, in turn, depends on individual views, which will be influenced by personal, professional, cultural, religious and political values. We do not suggest that these influences can be eliminated, but doctors must be aware of how these affect their analysis of any situation. Doctors' ethical values must also be capable of justification, and doctors must be constantly aware that ethical judgements must be based on the particular circumstances of each case and that any decisions arrived at must involve appropriate explanation and negotiation with patients or guardians.

Key points

- The fundamental principles in medical ethics are justice, respect for persons and the duty to do good.
- Doctors' personal values will affect how they analyse and react to an ethical dilemma.
- An ethical dilemma requires that real choices exist between potential actions, and that the differences between these actions are important.
- A satisfactory solution to an ethical dilemma should have consequences which do not conflict with the values of the doctor, patient or society.
- Patients must be fully involved in any (negotiated) solution.

References

Brody, H. (1981). *Ethical Decisions in Medicine*, 2nd edn., p. 10. Boston: Little, Brown and Company.

Downie, R. S. and Calman, K. C. (1994). *Healthy Respect. Ethics in Health Care*, 2nd edn., p. 12. Oxford: Oxford University Press.

Gillon, R. (1986a). *Philosophical Medical Ethics*, pp. 116–17. Chichester: John Wiley & Sons.

Gillon, R. (1986b). *Philosophical Medical Ethics*, p. 1. Chichester: John Wiley & Sons.

Johnson, A. G. (1990a). *Pathways in Medical Ethics*, p. 20. London: Edward Arnold.

Johnson, A. G. (1990b). *Pathways in Medical Ethics*, p. 94. London: Edward Arnold.

Johnson, A. G. (1990). *Pathways in Medical Ethics*, p. 97–8. London: Edward Arnold.

Johnson, A. G. (1990). *Pathways in Medical Ethics*, p. 111. London: Edward Arnold.

Price, D. (1996). Lessons for health care rationing from the case of Child B. *British Medical Journal*, 312, 167–9.

Thompson, I. E. (1987). Fundamental ethical principles in health care. *British Medical Journal*, 295, 1461.

Appendix

Suggested response to Example 2

Issues which need to be considered are the patient's 'right' to a smear, respect for the patient, her wishes and her autonomy, the equity of repeat smears when a smear is 'not indicated', and the good and harm which may arise from performing this smear.

Potential courses of action

1. The doctor could refuse to perform a smear more frequently than every 3 years for a woman with no special indication for a more frequent smear and who is at low risk of cervical carcinoma.
2. The doctor could perform a cervical smear whenever the patient requests one.

If morbidity and mortality from cervical carcinoma are to be reduced, all women must be offered a cervical smear at regular intervals. It is more important to perform 3-yearly smears on all women rather than to perform smears more frequently on those who inappropriately request one (justice). It is important to avoid frequent, unnecessary smears so that the laboratory services are not overloaded by large numbers of smears that are unlikely to be abnormal, and reports on abnormal smears are not delayed (non-maleficence). Performing the smear will relieve the patient's anxiety, reassure her and, in the very unlikely event of her developing cervical neoplasia since her last smear, it would be detected and treated early (beneficence). Performing the smear will protect the relationship between the doctor and the patient (beneficence), but encourage inappropriate use of limited resources (maleficence).

A doctor's decision on which course of action to take will depend on how that doctor weights these consequences. If preservation of the relationship with the patient is all important, the doctor will accept the second course of action and perform the smear. If the doctor feels that this patient's smear will delay other women's results unnecessarily, the request may be refused. However, neither of these courses of action may satisfy the doctor's values. In this event, the potential course of action (1) could be modified, perhaps to:

'The doctor could refuse to perform NHS smears more frequently than every 3 years for women with no indication for a smear or who are at low risk of cervical carcinoma.'

This provides for the benefits of performing the smear and avoids the disadvantage of the first course of action, if the patient can afford to pay for a smear. However, because it is dependent on ability to pay, this cannot be a general solution to the dilemma.

Suggested response to Example 3

Potential courses of action

1. The doctor could decide that there is nothing he can do.
2. The doctor could suggest to John that Sally must be told so that she is adequately diagnosed and treated.
3. The doctor could honour John's insistence on confidentiality by investigating and treating Sally by subterfuge; for example, by pretending that 'more tests' are required to investigate the couple's subfertility.
4. The doctor could suggest that John tells Sally he has a 'minor infection' that may be transmitted during intercourse, and that she needs to be examined to make sure she does not have it.

John has the right to expect that the confidentiality of his diagnosis will be respected and not divulged to anyone. Sally should be told the truth about why any investigations are performed or treatment is administered, otherwise her consent will be neither informed nor valid and therefore any investigation and treatment will infringe her autonomy. The principle of beneficence requires that Sally be properly treated, but also that their marriage is not damaged unnecessarily.

If the doctor decides to do nothing, Sally may be harmed by his inaction. The consequences of telling Sally that she may have a sexually transmitted disease are that she will be properly diagnosed and treated and her autonomy will have been respected. John's autonomy, however, will have been violated, and the relationships between John and Sally and the doctor and John damaged. If Sally is investigated by subterfuge her consent is invalid, since any examination performed would be an assault; John's autonomy and the marriage will have been protected. The 'half truth' about the minor infection will still infringe Sally's autonomy and, if she has a chlamydial infection, she has the right to know not only what the diagnosis is but, if she asks, what it means. However, this does not require the doctor to tell her about John's infidelity.

This case illustrates that there may not be a single 'right' answer in an ethical dilemma.

10

Clinical problem-solving and patient management: some practical challenges

Gary E. Aram and Robin C. Fraser

This chapter offers you some practical opportunities for self-testing the extent to which you have become familiar with the consultation competences described in this book.

The first part of the chapter sets out a variety of clinical scenarios typical of those that you would be likely to encounter in any general practice. They contain a mix of problems that include physical, social and psychological dimensions and involve patients of various ages. Each scenario is followed by specific questions, which you are invited to answer *before* comparing your answers with those set out in the second half of the chapter. *You will be given new information as the scenario progresses. Accordingly, these exercises will be more useful to you if you do not read this information until you have completed the previous question(s).* Doing so will affect your answer(s), usually by focusing your thought processes on a particular area, which will often be an inappropriate restriction. The answers that we have provided are meant to represent a reasonable way of dealing with the particular scenarios, but they are not meant to represent the *only* way.

You will notice that you will be asked to give reasons and explanations for your responses to the various questions. This is because we want to encourage you to articulate your reasoning processes as well as test your ability to arrive at the 'correct' actions and solutions. It is through an understanding of the strengths and weaknesses of your own reasoning processes that you will improve your ability to react to the wide range of future clinical challenges which you will inevitably encounter as a doctor.

Scenario 1

Jan Matthews is a university student, aged 21 years. She attends infrequently for minor illness and holiday immunizations.

Today she enters looking well, but appears worried. She tells you she has had lower abdominal pain 'off and on' for some months, and that it 'has got a lot worse' over the last month. It is now present 'almost all the time'.

Question 1

What are your initial diagnostic hypotheses? Explain how you arrived at these.

Question 2

What questions would you want to ask to test your respective hypotheses? Explain how the questions might help you.

Scenario 2

Mrs Foxton consults you as she is having difficulty with her daughter Melanie, aged 16 years, who has been staying out late at night and was brought home drunk from a party three nights previously. You offer to see Mrs Foxton and Melanie together to discuss the situation, but Mrs Foxton is not convinced Melanie will agree.

Three weeks later, Melanie comes to see you complaining of a vaginal discharge.

Question 3

What are your initial diagnostic hypotheses? Explain how you arrived at these.

Question 4

What questions would you want to ask to test your respective hypotheses? Explain how the questions might help you.

(*Answer questions before proceeding.*)

Melanie tells you that over the last month she has had regular unprotected sexual intercourse with her new boyfriend, aged 17 years. Her period, which is usually regular, is now 2 days late. She has had no previous sexual partner and no other symptoms of pregnancy. Her discharge is white and itchy, and vaginal examination strongly suggests candida infection.

Question 5

How would you manage Melanie at this consultation?

(*Answer question before proceeding.*)

A week later Melanie comes to see you for the result of her pregnancy test, which is negative.

Question 6

You confirm the result with Melanie. What other issues might you discuss at this consultation?

Scenario 3

Mrs Shilton brings her daughter Eve, aged 18 months, to the surgery and tells you, 'Eve has been unwell for 3 days with a runny nose and a cough. Last night she didn't sleep at all because she seemed to be feverish and in pain'. Further history reveals no more useful information.

Question 7

What are your initial diagnostic hypotheses? Explain how you arrived at these.

Question 8

What examination would you now perform to test your respective hypotheses? Explain how your chosen examination might help you.

Scenario 4

Your next patient is Mr Charnwood, a retired postman aged 66 years. He has been healthy all his life and rarely attends any doctor. He tells you that over the previous 6 weeks he has been increasingly short of breath.

Question 9

What are your initial diagnostic hypotheses? Explain how you arrived at these.

Question 10

What questions would you want to ask to test your respective hypotheses? Explain how the questions might help you.

(*Answer questions before proceeding.*)

From your history, you learn that Mr Charnwood's dyspnoea is mainly on exertion and his exercise tolerance has gradually diminished to 100 m. More recently he has noticed dyspnoea when lying flat in bed, and he now uses three pillows, but he has had no paroxysmal nocturnal dyspnoea (PND). He has no wheeze. He has previously been well apart from some pain in his knees that he assumes to be due to his previous occupation. Ibuprofen from the pharmacist has always helped this symptom, and has not given him any indigestion. On checking his records you notice he had a blood pressure reading of 180/100 5 years previously. He was asked to return for further readings but did not attend. There is no further significant history.

Question 11
What are your hypotheses now? Explain how you arrived at these.

Question 12
What examination would you now perform to test your respective hypotheses? Explain how your examination might help you.

(*Answer questions before proceeding.*)

On examination Mr Charnwood looks well, is not dyspnoeic at rest (respiratory rate 15 per minute) and shows no evidence of clinical anaemia. His pulse is regular at 80 beats per minute. His blood pressure is 200/110; there is evidence of cardiomegaly but no cardiac murmurs, and the fundi show arteriovenous nipping. Auscultation of the chest reveals bilateral fine basal crepitations.

Question 13
What are your hypotheses now? Explain how you arrived at these.

Question 14
How would you manage Mr Charnwood at this consultation?

Scenario 5

Mrs Eaves, aged 23 years, has been married to a lorry driver for 1 year. She had her second child, Ryan, 5 weeks previously after an un-complicated pregnancy and labour. She attends today with Debbie, her other child (aged 2 years), and Ryan. Both look rather untidy. Debbie has a leaking nappy and Ryan has been crying in his pushchair since they arrived. She asks you to look at Ryan, saying, 'I don't think he has been right for the last few days'.

Question 15
What are your initial diagnostic hypotheses? Explain how you arrived at these.

Question 16
What questions would you want to ask to test your respective hypotheses? Explain how the questions might help you.

(*Answer questions before proceeding.*)

You learn the baby is feeding well at 4-hourly intervals and has no specific symptoms, but Mrs Eaves tells you that he seems to be crying a lot.

Question 17
What are your hypotheses now? Explain how you arrived at these.

Question 18
What examination would you now perform to test your respective hypotheses? Explain how your examination might help you.

(*Answer questions before proceeding.*)

Ryan appears well. His crying settles as you handle him, and there are no abnormal findings. As you explain this to Mrs Eaves she admits to feeling depressed since the delivery, with loss of appetite, early morning waking, crying, loss of interest and exhaustion. She recognizes she is not coping, although she has some help from her mother. Her husband has offered to take time off work, but she feels guilty about this. There is no suggestion of any risk of harm to the children or herself.

Question 19
How would you manage Mrs Eaves at this consultation?

Scenario 6

Mrs Walters comes to see you with Debbie, her daughter (aged 7 years), whom you see about four times a year. She is usually a healthy though overweight child, and mostly presents with minor upper respiratory tract infections (URTI). Mrs Walters asks you to check Debbie as she has been complaining of abdominal pain almost every morning for the past 4 weeks. Debbie does not look unwell.

Question 20
What are your initial diagnostic hypotheses? Explain how you arrived at these.

Question 21
What questions would you want to ask to test your respective hypotheses? Explain how the questions might help you.

Scenario 7

Frank Shearsby, a recently married bricklayer aged 27 years, consults you complaining of low back pain which came on after lifting a heavy load at work the previous day. He is usually well and has consulted you only a few times in the past for minor illnesses. Examination indicates tenderness over both sacro-iliac joints, but there is no sciatic radiation. A diagnosis of simple back strain is made, and paracetamol + codeine compound is given. After 3 weeks there is little apparent improvement in his condition. The history and examination are still compatible with a simple back strain, and you explain this to him. Mr Shearsby is worried it could be something more serious, and asks if you could refer him to a specialist.

Question 22
What factors do you think could have increased Mr Shearsby's concern?

Question 23
How would you respond to Mr Shearsby's request for a referral?

(*Answer questions before proceeding.*)

Mr Shearsby tells you a colleague at work had sciatica, was off work for 9 months, and that he ultimately required surgery before he improved.

Question 24
How would you manage Mr Shearsby at this consultation?

Scenario 8

Miss Jennifer Sharnford, aged 38 years, is a sales director with a national clothing company. She attends only very occasionally and has no significant previous medical history. She plans to marry in 2 months' time and is looking forward to a fortnight's honeymoon in Kenya and Tanzania. Following this she wants to start a family, but thought she 'ought to come for a check-up' first.

Question 25
Identify the most useful preventive opportunities which are present in this consultation, and explain how you would proceed to act on them.

Scenario 9

Richard Whetstone comes to see you. He is a teacher aged 40 years, previously healthy, and married with two children aged 10 and 13 years. He complains of a cough of 2 weeks' duration, but in the past few days he has 'coughed up some blood'.

Question 26
What are your initial diagnostic hypotheses? Explain how you arrived at these.

Question 27

What questions would you want to ask to test your respective hypotheses? Explain how the questions might help you.

(Answer questions before proceeding.)

You learn that Mr Whetstone's cough is accompanied by green sputum and fever. The haemoptysis is dark and it has occurred several times. Yesterday he coughed up around 10 ml of blood in one bout. He has smoked 30 cigarettes per day for over 20 years. There are no other significant features in the history.

Question 28

What are your hypotheses now? Explain how you arrived at these.

Question 29

What examination would you now perform to test your respective hypotheses? Explain how your examination might help you.

(Answer questions before proceeding.)

Examination reveals some crepitations at the right base. You decide to order a chest X-ray, which shows a right hilar shadow strongly suggestive of carcinoma of the lung. Mr Whetstone returns to see you for the results of the X-ray.

Question 30

How would you manage Mr Whetstone at this consultation?

(Answer question before proceeding.)

You refer Mr Whetstone to a chest physician. The lesion is found to be an inoperable, anaplastic, undifferentiated adenocarcinoma of the lung. Mr Whetstone is made aware of the diagnosis and returns home to his wife and two children.

Question 31

List the problems that may arise now and in the future.

Scenario 10

Mrs Woodhouse is a nursing auxiliary, aged 45 years. She is generally fit although somewhat overweight (body mass index 31.6), and she smokes 10 cigarettes per day. For the past 3 years she has suffered from menorrhagia. Examination is difficult in view of her obesity, but reveals no abnormal findings. You decide to refer her for investigations and advice on management.

Mrs Woodhouse consults you again, having seen the gynaecologist the previous week. He performed a hysteroscopy (which she was told was normal), recommended a hysterectomy and placed her on the waiting list. You have not yet received the outpatient letter. Mrs Woodhouse says to you, 'I was a bit surprised to be told I needed a hysterectomy. My friend with similar symptoms had an endometrial ablation and has been fine since, but the gynaecologist said it probably wouldn't be successful and it wasn't a procedure he did anyway'.

Question 32
What ethical issues arise in this case, and what problems should be discussed with Mrs Woodhouse at this consultation?

(*Answer question before proceeding.*)

Mrs Woodhouse tells you that she understands the options available, but doesn't want a hysterectomy. She feels she could live with her heavy periods if there was no other option. She would find a major operation difficult in view of various family commitments. She asks you if you could 'prescribe something to help' or refer her to a specialist who may consider endometrial ablation.

Question 33
How would you now manage Mrs Woodhouse at this consultation?

Scenario 11
John Sutton, aged 29 years, has been married for 3 years. He consults you for the first time after having seen the practice nurse the previous week for a new patient check. He has been previously healthy apart from mild eczema, and was told to see you to organize his repeat prescription for a steroid cream. The following data were entered by the nurse:

- Occupation   printer
- Family history   father myocardial infarction (MI) aged 55 years
- Allergies   Nil
- Smoking   10 cigarettes a day for 10 years
- Alcohol   6 units weekly
- Body   mass index 23
- Blood pressure   130/80
- Urinalysis   negative for glucose and protein
- Immunizations   all up to date

You confirm he has mild eczema, which is satisfactorily controlled with the occasional use of 1% hydrocortisone cream. You organize a repeat prescription for this.

Question 34
Identify the most useful preventive opportunities that are present at this consultation, and explain how you would proceed to act on them.

Answers to questions

Scenario 1 – Jan Matthews

Question 1
(What are your initial diagnostic hypotheses? Explain how you arrived at these.)

Pre-diagnostic interpretations
Although the problem is chronic and getting worse, serious pathology is unlikely because she looks well despite several months of pain. However, she is an infrequent attender and today looks concerned, suggesting she is either worried by her symptoms or is finding they are beginning to interfere with her life. Her age would suggest she is in her final year at university with approaching examinations. Accordingly, the most likely cause of her chronic lower abdominal pain could be either physical (gastrointestinal or gynaecological) or psychological.

Hypotheses
Most likely   *Less likely*
Irritable bowel syndrome (IBS)   Pelvic inflammatory disease (PID)
Anxiety state

IBS is common in young females, is non-serious, and you would expect the patient to look well. The pain would be of a recurrent chronic nature, and could be aggravated by the stress of examinations.

There may be other worries in her life, e.g. boyfriend difficulties, which would induce anxiety and may present as abdominal pain. Her abdominal pain may itself have induced concerns of serious underlying disease that may then have exacerbated it.

PID is possible in a young sexually active female, but you are as yet unaware of her sexual history and any associated infection.

Question 2
(What questions would you want to ask to test your respective hypotheses? Explain how the questions might help you.)

First, clarify the presenting symptom of abdominal pain. This will determine whether it is the same pain throughout, despite becoming worse. If not, you may be required to develop new hypotheses.

1. *Site +/− radiation.* Generalized (lower) abdominal pain would support IBS and anxiety. Pelvic pain would be more supportive of PID. Radiation is unlikely to be a feature of either.
2. *Quality.* A colicky pain would support IBS, a more constant pain would support anxiety and a dragging, constant pain would support PID.
3. *Severity.* This is likely to be very variable in both IBS and anxiety. The pain of IBS would tend to be either mild or moderate, whilst that of anxiety would be proportionate to the severity of the anxiety. PID is usually of mild to moderate severity, although it can, rarely, mimic an acute abdomen.
4. *Periodicity.* You already know the duration and progression of symptoms. You now need to look for alterations within the day or week. Association with food/mealtimes supports IBS, times of increased stress would exacerbate the pain of anxiety, whilst increased pain related to menstruation would support PID.
5. *Precipitating, exacerbating or relieving factors.* Is the patient aware of any change that has coincided with the onset or increase of the pain? Stress would aggravate or precipitate the pain of IBS and anxiety, whilst defecation might ease the pain in IBS. Sexual intercourse would aggravate PID pain (deep dyspareunia), whilst the coincidence of pain onset with a new partner might suggest the start of an infection.
6. *Associated features.* A variable bowel habit alternating between constipation and diarrhoea associated with abdominal distension, flatus or mucus per rectum supports IBS. Other symptoms of anxiety include disturbed sleep, palpitations and reduced appetite. Generalized systemic upset would suggest PID, which would be further supported by a fever, change in menstrual cycle or vaginal discharge.
7. *Confirm the patient's concerns and reason for attendance today.* She might be finding the pain unbearable as it is now continuous. However, there may be underlying concerns about what the pain might signify, e.g. cervical cancer, that you would be unlikely to address unless mentioned by the patient. Ask an open question, e.g. 'You look concerned about the pain, is there anything in particular worrying you?'

It would then be appropriate to search for specific associated features relating to each hypothesis still being considered. In doing so, you would need to indicate to the patient the reasons for your particular line of enquiry *(signalling)*, thereby gaining implied consent to continue.

IBS is recognized to have a strong psychological component. You therefore need to explore psychological issues and their effects with appropriate sensitivity. Areas of enquiry would include her studies (remember she is probably nearing her final examinations), relatives and partner(s).

This would also help identify underlying causes of anxiety. If these are not forthcoming, you need to ask specifically about particular symptoms of anxiety.

To diagnose PID you would need to take a sexual history, including previous and present partners who may have put her at potential risk. Establishing her method of contraception (if relevant) is important, as only barrier methods offer protection against PID.

Scenario 2 – Mrs Foxton and Melanie

Question 3
(What are your initial diagnostic hypotheses? Explain how you arrived at these.)

Pre-diagnostic interpretations
Mrs Foxton has indicated that Melanie might be sexually active and may have been at risk of unprotected sex when drunk. However, it is important not to break confidentiality and declare this knowledge to Melanie without Mrs Foxton's permission.

The acute onset of a vaginal discharge therefore raises the possibility of a sexually transmitted disease (STD), but we should still consider other infective causes of vaginal discharge. Melanie might also be worried about the risk of pregnancy or STD.

Hypotheses

Most likely	*Less likely*
1. Vaginitis:	Retained foreign body, e.g. tampon
(a) Non-sexually transmitted disease:	Physiological
(NSTD)	Ticket of admission
– candida	
– gardnerella	
(b) Sexually transmitted disease (STD):	
– trichomonas	
– chlamydia	
– gonorrhoea	
2. Pregnancy	

Candida (the commonest vaginal infection) and gardnerella are not specifically related to sexual intercourse, but if Melanie is sexually active the other three conditions need to be considered.

If Melanie is sexually active, you need to ascertain if she has been using contraception. A sheath would offer some protection from a STD and from pregnancy, depending on its correct usage – which could be in doubt based on her mother's story. Pregnancy or recent onset of sexual activity will increase the normal physiological discharge.

A retained tampon is not unusual, and may have been inserted and forgotten whilst she was drunk.

Melanie might be anxious in case she has contracted a STD or is pregnant, and may be requiring reassurance. This could also be a ticket of admission to discuss contraception or a relationship problem that she is unable to discuss with her mother.

Question 4

(What questions would you want to ask to test your respective hypotheses? Explain how the questions might help you).

Firstly clarify the presenting symptom.

1. *Characteristics* of the vaginal discharge will help to differentiate between the different causes:
   a. Candida: white, cottage cheese-like and itchy
   b. Gardnerella: grey-brown, fishy smell and itchy
   c. Trichomonas: profuse, frothy green-brown, offensive, itchy and sore
   d. Chlamydia: mild discharge and irritation – may be asymptomatic
   e. Gonorrhoea: light green and offensive
   f. Pregnancy: clear, but heavier than usual physiological discharge
   g. Retained foreign body: brown and offensive.
2. *Duration.* A short duration (e.g. < 2 weeks) increases the likelihood of STD. If present only since her last period, a retained tampon is possible.
3. *Severity.* Does it only lightly stain her underwear, or does she need to use a pad or tampon? A heavier discharge would be expected with gardnerella, trichomonas, gonorrhoea or retained tampon.
4. *Precipitating, exacerbating or relieving factors.* A physiological discharge would be worse premenstrually.
5. *Associated features.* Candida is usually associated with a pruritis. Gardnerella and trichomonas may also be associated with pruritis.
6. *Previous history.* Is there a history of previous similar discharge? This is commonly seen with candida infections.

Depending on the responses to the above, it may now be appropriate to search for specific features relating to remaining hypotheses.

- Ask if Melanie uses tampons
- Confirm if Melanie is sexually active or not – if so, ascertain:
  - her sexual behaviour, i.e. one night relationships or a regular boyfriend? Is she aware of her partner's sexual history?
  - whether she is using contraception, its form and if she is using it reliably
  - if she has any specific concerns or fears.

The latter question will help to assess the risk of STD or pregnancy and her contraceptive needs.

The fact that she is presenting with a vaginal discharge will indicate the relevance of these intimate questions, but they need to be asked with sensitivity and when a reasonable rapport has developed. At no time should you indicate your prior knowledge, which was obtained from her mother, as this will damage any trusting relationship and break confidentiality.

If Melanie has been sexually active (especially if she has been using an unreliable form of contraception or none at all), you need to check her last menstrual period (LMP) and normal menstrual cycle to assess the possibility of pregnancy. If her period is delayed, other symptoms of pregnancy should be sought, e.g. breast tenderness, nausea or frequency of micturition.

Finally, it is important to give Melanie an opportunity to discuss other issues that may have made her present today, e.g. contraceptive needs or relationship problems. She will probably be encouraged by an empathic response from someone who appears to understand her needs and is willing to listen to her as an adult.

Question 5
(How would you manage Melanie at this consultation?)

Use *RAPRIOP* to structure your management.

1. *Reassurance and explanation.* Tell Melanie that she probably has 'thrush', a common, non-serious infection that is not sexually transmitted and is easily treated.
2. Discuss the possibility of an early pregnancy and her attitude to this. Explain it is not unusual for her period to be delayed, especially if she has been worried about the risk she has taken. Nevertheless, suggest to her that you think it would be wise to arrange a pregnancy test as a precaution.
3. *Advice.* Discuss the risk of sexually transmitted disease and her need for contraception. Check her understanding first and inform as appropriate, being careful not to appear as a 'parent' telling a 'child' how to behave. Offer advice on safe sex and the use of condoms. Does she in addition require an oral contraceptive? If so, first exclude contraindications such as migraine, thrombosis and hypertension, and check smoking status.
4. *Prescription.* Issue a prescription for clotrimazole pessaries 500 mg inserted vaginally at night, or an oral antifungal such as fluconazole 150 mg. If requested the combined oral contraceptive, e.g. microgynon 30, could be prescribed now or at a follow-up consultation, to be commenced at the start of her next period if the pregnancy test is negative.

5. *Investigation.* Arrange a pregnancy test.
6. *Observation.* Arrange to review Melanie with the results of her test.
7. *Prevention.* Melanie will require a cervical smear, but this would be better left for the follow-up consultation. Melanie will still be concerned regarding a possible pregnancy, and therefore unlikely to concentrate on any advice offered.

Question 6
(You confirm the result with Melanie. What other issues might you discuss at this consultation?)

- Offer help with emotional problems relating to her boyfriend, parents or peers. Encourage Melanie to talk to her mother, but be careful not to break confidentiality.
- If she smokes, offer advice on stopping, especially if she is to commence the oral contraceptive. You will need to explain the risks to her. If she is willing to stop, let her know she can obtain support by visiting the practice nurse. If she commences the oral contraceptive you will have the opportunity to review this at her follow-up.
- It might be worth asking about drug abuse if an appropriate opportunity arises. However, it is important not to try to tackle too many issues in one consultation and risk damaging the doctor–patient relationship.
- Arrange to see her after 3 months to assess progress on the oral contraceptive if prescribed.

Scenario 3 (Mrs Shilton and family)

Question 7
(What are your initial diagnostic hypotheses? Explain how you arrived at these.)

Pre-diagnostic interpretation
This is an acute illness and probably infective in origin in view of the likely fever and presenting respiratory symptoms. You assume the mother is concerned because after 3 days Eve is getting worse, as she is now in pain and is obviously unwell.

Hypotheses
Most likely	*Less likely*
Upper respiratory tract infection (URTI)	Lower respiratory tract infection (LRTI)
Otitis media	Meningitis

The history suggests an initial URTI, which may have progressed to an episode of otitis media or a LRTI.

Otitis media would frequently cause pain, which would be absent in a LRTI, and it should be noted that Mrs Shilton has interpreted Eve's symptoms as being related to pain. The absence of any difficulty with Eve's breathing would again make a LRTI less likely.

Meningitis is not common, but it is essential not to miss it as it may not present with classical features at this age. It may well present a few days after an URTI, and remember, Eve is now unwell.

Question 8
(What examination would you now perform to test your respective hypotheses? Explain how your chosen examination might help you).

Begin with a general examination, then examine the throat, ears, lungs and check for neck stiffness, photophobia and rash.

General examination
Does Eve look ill? Is she drowsy, irritable or miserable? If she is, you are more likely to consider meningitis. A high temperature would support otitis media, LRTI or meningitis. A tachycardia is non-specific, but would support a fever or more serious illness.

Specific examination
To confirm or refute your hypotheses, a specific examination should now be performed in an order which the child finds least upsetting.

Photophobia and neck stiffness should be looked for, but are not always present in cases of meningitis at this age. It is mandatory to look for the petechial rash of meningococcal septicaemia, but be aware of the possibility of a non-specific rash being present with viral infections.

A raised respiratory rate, possibly with the use of accessory muscles, supports a LRTI. Percussion of the chest may be decreased in the presence of a pneumonic LRTI and there may also be added crepitations on auscultation. Rhonchi would be heard if it were a bronchiolitic LRTI.

A dull, bulging, red tympanic membrane would confirm the diagnosis of otitis media.

Look for tonsillar and anterior cervical lymphadenopathy, then examine the throat for signs of inflammation +/− tonsillar exudates and post nasal drip to confirm an URTI.

Scenario 4 (Mr Charnwood)
Question 9
(What are your initial diagnostic hypotheses? Explain how you arrived at these.)

Pre-diagnostic interpretations

As Mr Charnwood is an infrequent attender who is rarely ill, he must be given particular attention. The system most likely to be involved in sub-acute, progressive dyspnoea in a man of this age is the cardio-vascular system, although respiratory and haemopoietic systems are less likely possibilities.

Hypotheses

Most likely   *Less likely*

Left ventricular failure (LVF) due to: Iron deficiency anaemia

a. ischaemic heart disease (IHD)   Asthma

b. hypertensive heart disease

The most likely cardiovascular cause is either ischaemic or hypertensive heart disease leading to LVF, but Mr Charnwood rarely attends doctors and may have undiagnosed hypertension. A (silent) myocardial infarction (MI) occurring 6 weeks previously also needs to be considered.

Anaemia may present with progressive dyspnoea over a 6-week period; however a cause for any anaemia would then need to be sought. The most likely cause in Mr Charnwood's case would be occult blood loss from the gastrointestinal tract (e.g. an undiagnosed bowel lesion or a gastric/duodenal ulcer, which could be due to self-medication).

Late onset asthma is a possibility, although it usually presents with a cough +/− wheeze and there is often a previous (intermittent) history.

Chronic respiratory problems such as chronic obstructive airways disease and fibrosing alveolitis would be highly unlikely with such a short history in a previously well gentleman. If he had previously had difficulties with breathing, it would surely have interfered with his work as a postman and made him present earlier.

Question 10

(What questions would you want to ask to test your respective hypotheses? Explain how the questions might help you.)

Start by clarifying the presenting symptom, i.e. shortness of breath.

1. *Duration.* You already know that it is of 6 weeks' duration and increasing in severity.
2. *Onset.* Was it sudden, supporting a (silent) MI, or related to an environmental change, e.g. a new pet following his retirement. A more gradual onset would support your other hypotheses.
3. *Severity.* You already know it is getting worse, but you should establish his exercise tolerance. Severe LVF would be supported by the presence of PND.
4. *Periodicity.* Is it continuous or intermittent? If it is the latter, when does it come on? Asthma would be the only one of our hypotheses that varied significantly from day to day.

5. *Precipitating, exacerbating and relieving factors*. All hypotheses would be aggravated by exercise. LVF and anaemia would ease with rest, whilst asthma may not. LVF would be aggravated by lying down (orthopnoea) and eased by sitting up. Asthma may be triggered by even a mild respiratory infection, by cold air or proximity to a pet.

6. *Associated features*. LVF would be supported by pink frothy sputum and, if severe, by the presence of ankle swelling from a consequent right ventricular failure. IHD would almost always be accompanied by chest pain, although a silent MI can occur in the elderly. Other symptoms of anaemia would include tiredness. The presence of a dry cough or wheeze would support asthma, which would be even more strongly supported by the association of symptoms with a new pet.

You now need to search for specific features to support or refute your hypotheses.

- Check Mr Charnwood's notes for a record of any raised blood pressure readings.
- Does he have any relevant history not previously declared?
- Is there a family history of IHD, cerebrovascular disease, hyperlipidaemia or diabetes to support IHD? A history of smoking would also be supportive of IHD.
- Is there a history to suggest blood loss as a cause of anaemia? If there had been any frank bleeding per rectum or haematemesis, you would expect Mr Charnwood to have mentioned this. However, if tell him why you are asking questions relating to the gastrointestinal tract (which would otherwise appear unrelated or worrying), he will be able to help you look for clues (*signalling*).
- Is there a history of dyspepsia, non-steroidal drug use or excessive alcohol intake to support peptic ulcer disease? If so, establish whether or not he has black stools, suggesting blood loss.

Question 11
(What are your hypotheses now? Explain how you arrived at these.)

Hypotheses
Most likely   *Less likely*
LVF due to: Iron deficiency anaemia
a. Hypertensive disease
b. IHD

One raised blood pressure reading is not diagnostic of hypertension, but it may well be higher now due to age-related atherosclerosis. Mr Charnwood may therefore have had untreated hypertension for several years, resulting in the development of LVF. The dyspnoea of LVF would be worse on exertion, and there is a history of orthopnoea, although no PND or frothy pink sputum.

There is no history of chest pain to support IHD, but a silent MI can still not be excluded.

Anaemia remains a possibility, particularly in view of his use of non-steroidal anti-inflammatory drugs. Any blood loss may be occult, but there is no history of dyspepsia. The cardiovascular system would be able to compensate for a gradual loss for some time, and vague symptoms may have gone unnoticed.

You can rule out asthma, as the dyspnoea has been gradually progressive over 6 weeks and asthma is not associated with orthopnoea. Additionally, there are no supporting respiratory symptoms of cough or wheeze.

Question 12
(What examination would you now perform to test your respective hypotheses? Explain how your examination might help you.)

Start with a general examination.

Is the patient dyspnoeic at rest or whilst speaking? Does he look ill? If so, the condition is severe. The presence of cyanosis would indicate severe LVF; however, if anaemic, cyanosis is unlikely. Check for clinical signs of anaemia by looking for pale mucous membranes, conjunctivae, palmar creases and nail beds. There may be evidence of glossitis or koilonychia if the anaemia is more chronic.

You should now seek definitive clinical signs to confirm or refute your hypotheses.

Check the pulse rate and rhythm. You would expect to find a sinus tachycardia. Hypertensive heart disease and IHD may produce various arrhythmias, most commonly atrial fibrillation (confirm by radial deficit) and supraventricular tachycardia. Occasionally heart block may occur.

Take the blood pressure. If raised:

1. Determine the presence or absence of cardiomegaly (an important prognostic sign) and, if present, auscultate for associated valvular lesions, e.g. mitral incompetence
2. Examine both fundi for signs of hypertensive retinopathy.

Check the respiratory rate to further assess severity and assist in monitoring progress. Auscultate for fine (usually bilateral) basal crepitations as evidence of pulmonary oedema due to LVF.

(There is no history of right-sided failure, therefore checking for ankle oedema, hepatomegaly and a raised jugular venous pressure would be inappropriate.)

If there is evidence to suggest anaemia due to gastrointestinal blood loss, abdominal and rectal examinations should be undertaken to check for masses and/or a black stool on the examination glove.

Question 13
(What are your hypotheses now? Explain how you arrived at these.)

Hypotheses
Most Likely   *Less likely*
LVF due to hypertensive heart disease   LVF due to IHD

Mr Charnwood's blood pressure is significantly raised. Presumably he has had long-standing hypertension that has resulted in cardiomegaly and LVF. The bilateral fine basal crepitations support the presence of LVF. It is still possible that he may also have had a silent MI as a consequence of hypertensive heart disease, which has precipitated LVF. As there are no clinical signs of anaemia this hypothesis can be discarded.

Question 14
(How would you manage Mr Charnwood at this consultation?)

Use *RAPRIOP* to structure your management.

1. *Reassurance and explanation.* Use language he will understand. Explain that his blood pressure is raised and that this is 'straining his heart'. As a consequence, some fluid is collecting in his lungs and making him breathless. Reassure him that you can control his blood pressure, clear the fluid and make him less breathless.
2. *Advice.* He should rest and avoid lying flat until his symptoms start improving on treatment. A low salt diet will help.
3. *Prescription.* An angiotensin-converting enzyme (ACE) inhibitor, e.g. Lisinopril initially 2.5 mg daily increasing over 2–4 weeks to a maintenance dose of 5–20 mg daily, will reduce his blood pressure and improve his LVF. He should be informed of the risk of hypotensive effects. A loop diuretic, e.g. frusemide 40 mg daily, may also be used, but beware of potentiating the hypotensive effects.
4. *Referral.* A referral would not be indicated at this stage.
5. *Investigation.* An ECG would confirm ventricular hypertrophy and exclude a previous MI. A chest X-ray would confirm cardiomegaly and pulmonary oedema, although an echocardiogram is the investigation of choice to confirm cardiomegaly. Urea and electrolytes should be performed to exclude renal failure since the use of an ACE inhibitor is envisaged.
6. *Observation.* Review in 1–2 weeks to monitor progress (including his blood pressure), check for drug side-effects, review investigations and consider increasing therapy. Advise Mr Charnwood to see you earlier if there is any deterioration in his symptoms.

7. *Prevention.* Although you have not seen Mr Charnwood for several years, it would be inappropriate to consider aspects of anticipatory care at this consultation. You already have considerable important information to impart, and you will be following him up when there will be more appropriate opportunities. (If Mr Charnwood had been a known smoker it would have been essential to advise him to stop.)

Scenario 5 (Mrs Eaves and family)

Question 15
(What are your initial diagnostic hypotheses? Explain how you arrived at these.)

Pre-diagnostic interpretation
There are likely to be considerable social and psychological influences in the consultation. Mrs Eaves was first pregnant when aged about 20 years, and you don't know whether Mr Eaves is the father. Shortly after her marriage she became pregnant again. As a lorry driver, her husband may work away from home a lot and therefore there may be little support at home. It appears Mrs Eaves is not able fully to look after herself and her children. It is only 5 weeks since she delivered, and Mrs Eaves will still be recovering.

The first question we should ask ourselves is, who is the patient? Is it Mrs Eaves or Ryan?

Nevertheless, it would be sensible to respond initially to Ryan's perceived needs, during which time you will be able to develop some insight into Mrs Eaves' state of mind and health.

Hypotheses
1. Ryan as the patient

Most likely	Less likely
Physical illness, e.g.:	Lower respiratory tract infection
– upper respiratory tract infection (URTI)	(LRTI)
– gastroenteritis	
– feeding problem	

2. Mrs Eaves as the patient

Most likely	Less likely
Not coping	Postnatal depression

You must first consider a physical problem, as this may have serious implications. A feeding problem is common at this age, whilst an URTI or gastroenteritis would be the most likely infective problem. However, more serious causes might need to be excluded, e.g. pneumonia.

It appears Mrs Eaves is not coping. She is possibly neglecting herself and her children (as witnessed by Debbie's leaking nappy and her lack of response to Ryan's distress). This would be aggravated by the likelihood of her husband not being able to offer significant support, and you are unaware of any additional potential support from relatives or friends. Additionally, Mrs Eaves may not be physically fit enough to cope with a baby aged 5 weeks and another young child.

Postnatal depression needs to be considered as it is serious and carries a considerable risk of either self-harm (suicide) or harm to the children. This consultation may represent a cry for help from Mrs Eaves.

Question 16
(What questions would you want to ask to test your respective hypotheses? Explain how the questions might help you.)

Start by asking Mrs Eaves to clarify what she means by, 'I don't think he has been right for the last few days', as this will enable you to generate more specific diagnostic hypotheses and help you to assess whether or not Ryan is physically unwell. It may also give Mrs Eaves an opportunity to express any fears or concerns she may have concerning Ryan or herself. It should also provide you with some insight into Mrs Eaves' state of mind.

If he is refusing feeds, lethargic or continuously irritable and crying you need to be concerned. Are there specific features to suggest a particular diagnosis? Is there a fever to support infection? A cough would support an URTI or LRTI infection. A runny nose would suggest an URTI, and rapid breathing would suggest pneumonia. Vomiting and diarrhoea would support gastroenteritis.

If, on the other hand, Ryan is satisfied by a feed and has no specific symptoms, it may be he is being fed insufficiently, which is more difficult to assess if he is being breast-fed. A review of his weight gain would help clarify this.

If Ryan does not appear unduly unwell, it would then be appropriate to explore Mrs Eaves' situation. Does she feel she is coping? Can she call on any social support? Depending on her response, it might be appropriate to ask sensitively about her attitude to the children. Does she have aggressive feelings towards them or fear she may harm them?

Loss of appetite, low mood, weeping and sleep disturbance, e.g. early morning wakening, would all indicate postnatal depression. If depression is suspected, suicidal/homicidal ideations *must* be checked for.

Question 17
(What are your hypotheses now? Explain how you arrived at these.)

Hypotheses

Most likely	*Less likely*
Maternal problem: not coping	Maternal problem: postnatal depression
	Physical illness of Ryan, e.g. URTI

A feeding problem is now unlikely. As Ryan seems to be well (apart from his crying), a physical illness is less likely but cannot yet be excluded. A serious physical disease is virtually ruled out, however.

A maternal problem is now more likely, as this would result in lack of attention to Ryan.

Question 18
(What examination would you now perform to test your respective hypotheses? Explain how your examination might help you.)

You need to confirm that Ryan is physically well by performing a general examination. Ask Mrs Eaves to undress him, and observe her behaviour with him to assess any evidence of inadequate maternal bonding.

Does Ryan quieten on handling? Does he look well? Is Ryan afebrile? If so, a significant illness is highly unlikely.

Confirm Ryan has been feeding adequately by looking for signs of dehydration. A sunken fontanelle or eyes, dry mouth and loss of skin turgor would confirm this.

If Ryan looks well, you should check for signs of abuse.

If, surprisingly, Ryan did show signs of a physical illness, you would need to re-rank your hypotheses or generate new hypotheses.

Question 19
(How would you manage Mrs Eaves at this consultation?)

Mrs Eaves has six core symptoms of depression that have been present for more than 2 weeks. This confirms the diagnosis of clinical depression.

Management should be based on *RAPRIOP*. To ensure compliance, negotiation of the management with Mrs Eaves is very important.

1. *Reassurance and explanation.* Agree with Mrs Eaves that she is rather low at this time. Explain that she is suffering from postnatal depression, which is quite common and not surprising considering everything she has to cope with. Reassure her that it was correct to seek help at this stage, that treatment is indicated and that this should start making her feel better in a 'couple of weeks or so'.
2. *Advice.* Tell her that it would be better if her husband did take some time off work over the next couple of weeks to provide support whilst the treatment begins to work. Alternatively, is there any other potential help available from family or friends? Hopefully, by making this part of your recommended management plan you will reduce her level of guilt and give her permission to request assistance.
3. *Prescription.* An antidepressant is indicated. If Mrs Eaves is breast feeding, tricyclic antidepressants have no recognized contraindications (e.g. amitriptyline increased gradually to 150 mg daily); otherwise, selective serotonin re-uptake inhibitors may be prescribed (e.g.

fluoxetine 20 mg daily). Inform Mrs Eaves of the common side-effects of amitriptyline if prescribed, i.e. constipation, dry mouth and altered visual acuity; that treatment with either antidepressant is likely to be needed for a minimum of 6 months, and compliance with regular medication is important.

4. *Referral.* Requesting the health visitor to make a call would be appropriate in order to check on other areas of potential need. Practical problems could be addressed, the need for social support examined and advice on child care discussed. It would be inappropriate to refer to a psychiatrist at this stage.

5. *Observation.* Arrange to review progress at the postnatal appointment in 1 week to provide moral support. Advise that significant improvement will not be seen at this stage.

6. *Anticipatory care.* Inappropriate at this stage.

Scenario 6 (Mrs Walters and family)

Question 20
(What are your initial diagnostic hypotheses? Explain how you arrived at these.)

Pre-diagnostic interpretations
Abdominal pain in children is common and usually there is no serious underlying physical cause. Debbie looks well, which would support a non-serious cause, but Mrs Walters seems concerned and you will need to explore her anxieties. It is more likely there is an underlying psychological cause, since the pain occurs only in the morning.

Hypotheses
Most likely	Less likely
Anxiety	Ticket of admission
Constipation	Urinary tract infection

The fact the pain is occurring *only* in the mornings suggests an avoidance strategy in an otherwise well child. Perhaps Debbie has problems at school, which may be related to her being teased about her weight problem. There may be problems at home causing anxiety.

Constipation is a common problem, particularly if eating habits are poor (as is suggested by Debbie being overweight). This can cause intermittent abdominal pain in an otherwise well child, but is unlikely to occur only in the mornings.

UTIs are uncommon in children, but can present with vague and otherwise unexplained abdominal pain without specific urinary symptoms. If undiagnosed, permanent renal damage can ensue.

You need to establish why Mrs Walters has waited 4 weeks to bring Debbie to the doctor. Is she concerned about a specific problem such as a 'grumbling appendix', which may have been mentioned by a relative? Does she want to discuss another problem, such as marital difficulty, which she feels Debbie has become aware of and which she thinks might be causing her pain?

Question 21

(What questions would you want to ask to test your respective hypotheses? Explain how the questions might help you.)

You need to start by clarifying the presenting symptom of abdominal pain. You should first ask for Mrs Walters' opinion and then for Debbie's, who by this time should be more comfortable in the consultation and happier to talk. Be aware that a 7-year-old child may not give a clear history.

1. *Site +/− radiation.* A variable or central site would support anxiety. Left iliac fossa pain would support constipation, whilst suprapubic or loin pain could occur with a UTI. Radiation of the pain is unlikely to occur with any of the suspected conditions.
2. *Quality.* Constipation will tend to produce an intermittent colicky pain.
3. *Severity.* This is very subjective and difficult to assess in a child, but is unlikely to be severe in view of the delay in attending. You might ask, 'what does the pain stop you doing?'.
4. *Periodicity.* The fact that the pain occurs *only* in the morning suggests a psychological cause, e.g. the worries of going to school.
5. *Precipitating, exacerbating and relieving factors.* Pain related to anxiety would be present at times of stress and may have been precipitated by a significant change at school or home. Equally, symptoms would be less apparent whilst Debbie is enjoying herself, e.g. at weekends. The passage of hard, constipated motions is likely to produce local pain on defecation, which would be absent with the other conditions. Pain related to a UTI might also be accompanied by dysuria.
6. *Associated features.* A UTI would be supported if any of the classical urinary symptoms of fever, frequency, nocturia, dysuria and, more specifically in children, enuresis were present, although anxiety may also produce urinary frequency and enuresis.
7. *Confirm Mrs Walters' concerns and her reason for attendance today.* Ask open questions, e.g. 'Were you concerned about anything in particular when you asked me to check Debbie?' or, 'From what you have told me so far and after looking at Debbie, I doubt there is anything too serious going on. Before I examine her is there anything else I should know?' Hopefully this will clarify any concerns and give Mrs Walters an opportunity to discuss any underlying issues.

Depending upon the above history, it would then be appropriate to search for any additional but specific features relating to each hypothesis still being considered.

If it appears Debbie is anxious, a more detailed history of the school and home situation should be taken, e.g. bullying, teasing, marital unrest or illness in a relative. Other features of psychological problems should also be sought, e.g. demanding behaviour.

If Debbie appears to be constipated, a dietary history will be required in order to offer appropriate corrective advice.

If Mrs Walters has raised another issue, this should be pursued as appropriate.

Scenario 7 (Frank Shearsby)

Question 22
(What factors do you think could have increased Mr Shearsby's concern?)

As a bricklayer, Mr Shearsby has probably been unable to work for the last 3 weeks. This may have financial implications, or there may even be a risk he could lose his job. He may be concerned about his future fitness.

Presumably he has had muscle strains before that have improved over a few days. He may therefore have expected his back to be better by now. He might be worried that you may have made the wrong diagnosis, or fear he may have a more serious problem. Perhaps he knows of a relative or friend with a similar presentation, which turned out to have a serious underlying cause.

As the injury occurred at work, it is possible that he is seeking compensation.

Mr Shearsby's wife may be more concerned than he is, and she may have suggested he asks for a second opinion. The back pain may be affecting their marriage, particularly from a sexual aspect.

Question 23
(How would you respond to Mr Shearsby's request for a referral?)

You need to clarify his reasons for this request in order to respond appropriately. However, you should respect his right for a second opinion if this is clinically justifiable, and let him know that you are prepared to arrange this for him if you think it is warranted.

The use of open, reflective questions in a non-threatening manner might well encourage him to express his concerns. Such questions might include, 'You say you are worried it may be something more serious. What is it you are worried about?' and 'You have asked to see a specialist. What do you hope he will be able to do for you?'. Depending upon his response, more probing questions might be required to further explore his concerns.

Question 24

(How would you manage Mr Shearsby at this consultation?)

Further management should be based on *RAPRIOP*.

1. *Reassurance and explanation*. Having elicited Mr Shearsby's concerns, you should be able to reassure him that he does not have sciatica. Explain that sciatica involves the aggravation of the sciatic nerve and pain would be likely to extend/radiate down the leg with (possibly) signs of nerve involvement, which he does not have. It will then be necessary to explain to him:
   a. Why it is likely he still has a simple back strain, i.e. onset with lifting, localized tenderness
   b. That the duration of backache is difficult to predict accurately and that it could last for several weeks.
   You may have to counter some of his misconceptions regarding simple muscular strains and their duration.
2. *Advice*. You need to find out whether previous advice has been followed. Maintaining mobility is a crucial part of active back management. He should avoid bed rest or prolonged sitting, and needs to be made aware of correct posture. He should be shown how to bend and lift properly, especially as this may have precipitated his injury. Advice on suitable exercises could also be given. Be aware he may need certified absence from work.
3. *Prescription*. You should check that Mr Shearsby has been taking his prescribed medication. If so, you need to know if it has been adequate to allow him to remain mobile. Either one or a combination of the following drugs would be appropriate:
   a. A non-steroidal anti-inflammatory, e.g. ibuprofen 400 mg every 8 hours, which should be taken with food; alcohol should be avoided and he should be warned about potential dyspepsia
   b. A muscle relaxant, e.g. diazepam 5 mg every 8 hours for a few days only, although this may cause drowsiness.
4. *Referral*. This will depend upon the extent of Mr Shearsby's acceptance of your explanation and reassurance. Hopefully, it might be useful to negotiate by saying you would like him to give your suggested management plan a chance. Perhaps a physiotherapist could provide more specific advice and treatment. Agree to refer him to a specialist if his backache is not improving after another 2 weeks.
5. *Investigation*. Although an X-ray of the lumbar and sacral spine might aid reassurance, it is not usually helpful in cases of low back pain. You should therefore resist any request for or insistence on X-ray examination.

6. *Observation.* It would be appropriate to arrange a review of progress in 2–3 weeks, primarily to reassure Mr Shearsby that you acknowledge his concerns. You should point out that the need to refer can then be reassessed. Alternatively, if Mr Shearsby appears adequately reassured, you could leave him with an open appointment suggesting he returns if there is no progress.

7. *Prevention.* It is probably inappropriate to consider aspects of anticipatory care that are not related to his back problem in this consultation so as not to detract from your main message. Since he is an infrequent attender, however, you might decide to check his smoking habits, blood pressure and family history of cardiovascular disease at the follow up consultation.

Scenario 8 (Miss Jennifer Sharnford)

Question 25

(Identify the most useful preventive opportunities which are present at this consultation and explain how you would proceed to act on them.)

Since several opportunities present, there is a consequent risk of information overload. You should recognize that Miss Sharnford is an intelligent woman and present her with appropriate, clear and prioritized information. The use of explicit categorization, stating the most important points first and then summarizing (perhaps with the use of handouts/leaflets), are some of the communication skills you should employ.

The two main topics to be covered are foreign travel advice and pre-conception care.

Foreign travel advice

The most important aspects are protective immunizations and malaria prophylaxis. If you are unsure of the current requirements for Kenya and Tanzania (as is likely to be the case), consult an up-to-date information source. At the time of writing the requirements are as follows:

Recommended	*Sometimes recommended*
tetanus	diphtheria
polio	tuberculosis
hepatitis A	hepatitis B
typhoid	rabies
yellow fever	meningitis
malaria cover (proguanil + chloroquine)	

Her relative risk of exposure will need to be assessed in conjunction with current recommendations to enable the most appropriate regime to be identified. If she intends to stay in quality hotels and undertakes no high-risk activity, only those recommended requirements are indicated. Make it clear that malaria cover should commence 1 week prior to travel and continue for 4 weeks after her return. General health care advice should also be given, concentrating on the avoidance of mosquito bites. Provide her with the *Health Advice for Travellers* booklet, as it contains useful additional general advice on health care when abroad.

Pre-conception care

Miss Sharnford is aged 38 years and nulliparous; you should concentrate, therefore, on four main areas: counselling, lifestyle advice, appropriate physical examination and investigations.

1. *Counselling*
   a. The most important topic is the risk of foetal abnormality with increasing maternal age. Her views (and those of her future husband) on screening for neural tube defects and Down's syndrome should be ascertained. This should include their attitude and likely response if tests prove positive, particularly with reference to a potential termination of pregnancy. Advise her that commencing folic acid 400 µg daily now until the 12th week of pregnancy would reduce the risk of neural tube defects, and provide her with a prescription if required.
   b. Advise her to avoid pregnancy whilst taking antimalarials and, subsequently, to avoid unnecessary medication whilst trying to conceive. You are not aware of her current contraceptive method, but a barrier method would probably be optimal if she wishes to conceive in the near future.
2. *Lifestyle*
   a. You should elicit her dietary habits to ensure a balanced diet.
   b. Ask about her smoking and alcohol consumption, then advise accordingly.
3. *Examination*
   a. Assess her body mass index (BMI). If she is overweight, discuss the benefits of weight control both for herself and in view of a future pregnancy. Check her current eating habits and negotiate a modified diet sheet. Since follow-up usually improves patient response to diet, consider referral to a practice nurse or dietician.
   b. The blood pressure should be checked and follow-up readings carried out if necessary.
4. *Investigation*
   a. You should check she is up to date in respect of cervical cytology and, if this is not the case, she should make an appointment with the practice nurse to have a smear.
   b. Live vaccines should be avoided in pregnancy, including Rubella. Offer to check her Rubella status today so the vaccination can be given prior to conception if her immunity is low or absent.

Scenario 9 (Richard Whetstone)

Question 26
(What are your initial diagnostic hypotheses? Explain how you arrived at these.)

Pre-diagnostic interpretation
A 2-week cough in a previously healthy man aged 40 years suggests an infective non-life threatening cause. Although a local cause for hae-moptysis is possible, e.g. a congested throat in association with an upper respiratory tract infection (URTI), a more serious cause still needs to be considered.

Hypotheses

Most likely	*Less likely*
URTI	Carcinoma of the lung
Acute bronchitis	Tuberculosis (TB)

The most likely explanation is that he has an URTI with local damage to a congested blood vessel in the throat.

Acute bronchitis is often preceded by an URTI. It does not normally cause haemoptysis, but the repeated effort of coughing may cause a congested blood vessel to rupture.

Although young for carcinoma of the lung, you need to determine whether Mr Whetstone has any additional risk factors.

TB is less prevalent now, but since haemoptysis is an important symptom of this curable disease and his occupation would place large numbers of children at risk, it has to be excluded.

Question 27
(What questions would you want to ask to test your respective hypotheses? Explain how the questions might help you.)

You need to clarify the two presenting symptoms. First the cough.

1. *Duration* of the cough is known, i.e. 2 weeks.
2. *Periodicity.* How frequent is the cough? Repetitive coughing due to a ticklish/sore throat suggests an URTI.
3. *Precipitating, exacerbating or relieving factors.* Anaesthetic lozenges would ease the cough of an URTI.
4. *Associated features.* Is the cough productive? An irritant, bronchial, non-productive cough would support carcinoma of the lung. A pro-ductive cough with purulent sputum would support acute bronchitis, but we could not exclude an underlying carcinoma with secondary infection if the sputum were purulent. The colour of the sputum would be yellow or green in acute bronchitis, but typically straw-coloured in TB.

Next, clarify the haemoptysis. What is the colour of the haemoptysis? Bright blood would support URTI, whilst dark blood supports acute bronchitis, carcinoma of the lung and TB. A small quantity or streaks of blood would suggest an URTI or acute bronchitis. There would be more frequent and copious amounts of blood, possibly with clots, in carcinoma of the lung or TB.

The next step is to look selectively for further information to help confirm or refute your diagnostic hypotheses.

Start by offering an open question, e.g. 'Have you noticed anything else apart from the cough and blood?' or 'How have you otherwise been in yourself?'. Mr Whetstone is likely to be concerned himself and you need to elicit his fears and concerns. Ask an open question, e.g. 'Coughing up blood is obviously a concern to you, have you any particular thoughts about it?'.

If this fails to produce any significant answer, more specific questions are needed. Those related to carcinoma of the lung and TB would need to be asked sensitively.

A fever supports infection but night sweats specifically support TB. Dyspnoea would be present in all conditions except an URTI, but would be more rapid in onset in acute bronchitis. For dyspnoea to develop in carcinoma of the lung or TB, either collapse or consolidation of a lobe or a pleural effusion would have to be present and the patient would be 'ill'. In either case, the history would usually be longer.

A pleuritic pain could be due to either infection or malignant involvement of the pleura.

Significant weight loss supports carcinoma of the lung or TB.

Smoking would support acute bronchitis and carcinoma of the lung. Conversely, carcinoma of the lung is very unlikely in non-smokers. If he is a smoker, ask about daily consumption: the heavier the smoker the greater the risk of carcinoma of the lung.

Question 28
(What are your hypotheses now? Explain how you arrived at these.)

Hypotheses
Most Likely   *Less likely*
Acute bronchitis   Carcinoma of the lung
                                 Tuberculosis (TB)

The green sputum and fever support infection. The smoking history supports both acute bronchitis and carcinoma of the lung. You cannot exclude TB on this additional history, but an URTI can now be ruled out in view of the colour and quantity of haemoptysis and the sputum.

Question 29
(What examination would you now perform to test your respective hypotheses? Explain how your examination might help you.)

Start with a general examination. Does Mr Whetstone look ill or well? If he looks ill, a serious underlying cause is more likely. A fever will support infection. If Mr Whetstone does have either carcinoma of the lung or TB, you would be unlikely to find signs of weight loss, finger clubbing or lymphadenopathy with such a short history, but these should be looked for.

Specific examination of the respiratory system will help to confirm or refute your hypotheses. Palpate the trachea, which may be deviated towards an area of collapse due to malignancy or TB, but away from an effusion due to malignancy. Percuss the chest and listen for dullness, which would be present over an area of collapse or consolidation and may sound stony dull if an effusion is present. Auscultate to listen for crepitations (which would indicate infection), rhonchi (which may be caused by an obstruction due to malignancy) and a pleural rub (which may be present in both infection and malignancy).

Question 30
(How would you manage Mr Whetstone at this consultation?)

Carcinoma of the lung is a serious illness with a relatively poor prognosis. You would expect Mr Whetstone to be concerned regarding his symptoms, but he may not have seriously considered a diagnosis of cancer and its implications. The diagnosis may therefore be a major shock to him. We need to show empathy and build an effective doctor–patient relationship. Assess how much information to give, which will be dependent upon his responses. It will be important to use silence and proceed at his pace, checking at each stage whether he wishes to continue. We should also bear in mind that the diagnosis has not been confirmed, leaving the remote possibility that he may not actually have cancer. This element of doubt would allow a time of adjustment, from being a well man to having a potentially terminal illness, for Mr Whetstone and his family prior to further confirmatory investigations. You also need to consider at which stage we should involve his wife in the discussion. It may be appropriate to ask Mr Whetstone if he would like another appointment when his wife can be present. However, if he expresses a desire to hear all the information, it is of course his ethical right to be given it.

When asked for the results, it may be appropriate to begin by saying, 'I'm afraid the news isn't good'. Explain that a shadow has been found on the X-ray. If he asks what this means, admit that there is a possibility of cancer which needs to be excluded by further investigation. Check his understanding of the problem and any preconceptions he may have. Some of his beliefs or fears may need discussing.

Discussion regarding treatment and prognosis is probably best avoided at this stage until you have further information, but inform him that treatment options are available.

Explain to him that a referral to a chest physician needs to be arranged on an urgent basis, but confirm whether he is in agreement with this.

Allow Mr Whetstone time to adjust to the news, and give him the opportunity to ask any further questions.

Be prepared to discuss what he is going to say to his wife and what he expects her response to be.

Let him know you are going to support him during this difficult time. Arrange a further appointment to see him after he has been to the hospital, or earlier if indicated. He may wish to attend with his wife.

Question 31
(List the problems that may arise now and in the future.)

Use the triple diagnosis to structure your response. Remember you are the doctor to the whole family.

Short-term problems

1. Physical:
   a. Secondary infection
   b. Symptom control, e.g. pain.
2. Social:
   a. The loss of his job and consequent financial problems
   b. The need to make a will
   c. His wife's and children's reactions to his illness and their potential loss
   d. The coping ability of the family.
3. Psychological:
   a. Anger, shock and denial
   b. Anxiety about his future
   c. Depression.

Longer-term problems

1. Physical:
   a. Secondary infection
   b. Symptom control, e.g. cough, pain, dyspnoea
   c. Nursing help, e.g. pressure areas, toileting needs, personal hygiene.
2. Social:
   a. The ability of the family to cope
   b. A decision on the place of dying.
3. Psychological:
   a. Richard's (non)-acceptance of dying
   b. The family's ability to cope with bereavement.

Scenario 10 (Mrs Woodhouse)

Question 32
(What ethical issues arise in this case and what problems should be discussed with Mrs Woodhouse at this consultation?)

During this consultation we should remember we are hearing only one side of a reported conversation. Much may have been forgotten by the patient, due to the shock of being told unexpectedly that she needed a hysterectomy.

The following ethical issues need to be considered:

- *Beneficence/maleficence.* A doctor's first duty is to do no harm. You need to ask yourself if a hysterectomy is the current treatment of choice for Mrs Woodhouse. Would she be better to await a natural menopause and try various medical options to try and help control her periods, or to cope with her heavy periods but run the risk of developing anaemia? A hysterectomy would stop menorrhagia, but it is a major operation with associated risks and a prolonged postoperative recovery period. Laser ablation of the endometrium is a less invasive procedure, but she would run the risk of symptom recurrence.
- *Justice.* There should be equity for all patients in the availability of treatment options. Patients should not necessarily be restricted by the personal clinical preferences of particular doctors, including yourself, unless supported by research evidence.
- *Truth telling/patient autonomy.* The patient has the right to be adequately informed of potential options, given a balanced view of the risks and benefits involved, and invited to make a choice from these options.
- *Informed consent.* Mrs Woodhouse has been listed for a hysterectomy, but she may not be fully aware of or understand its consequences, e.g. operative complications and the possible need for hormone replacement therapy (HRT) if bilateral salpingo-oophorectomy is also performed.

Problems to be discussed
You need to understand Mrs Woodhouse's reasons for attendance, as this will focus the discussion. You should check that she understands the nature of the different options. It may be necessary to counter some false beliefs.

Is she wanting:

- a further explanation as to why a hysterectomy has been chosen?
- information about the operation and postoperative recovery period?
- information on the consequences of a hysterectomy, e.g. the effect on her sex life, the need for HRT, etc?

- a second opinion from a consultant, who may perform an endometrial ablation?
- to complain about the gynaecologist?

Question 33
(How would you now manage Mrs Woodhouse at this consultation?)

1. *Explain* there are various prescribed drugs you could try and, if these failed, you would be happy to refer her to another consultant requesting endometrial ablation if she so wished. Confirm that she is happy with this plan. Remind her that you have not yet received the consultant's letter and if this contains any new or conflicting information you may have to revise your advice. Confirm that you will write to the consultant informing him of her decision to cancel the operation.
2. *Prescription.* First-line therapy would involve issuing a non-steroidal anti-inflammatory drug (NSAID), e.g. mefenamic acid 500 mg three times a day, tranexamic acid 1–1.5 g three or four times a day or ethamsylate 500 mg four times a day, all to be taken during menstruation. Hormone therapy would be a later option. Inform Mrs Woodhouse that all these drugs can cause gastrointestinal upset, and that a NSAID is best taken with or after food.
3. *Investigation.* Check her last full blood count result and, if this was previously low and/or over 3 months old, repeat it. This will give an indication as to the severity of the menorrhagia and necessity for new or continuing iron therapy.
4. *Observation.* Review after three periods to consider continuing therapy if effective or changing to an alternative. Confirm you will contact her if necessary regarding the outpatient letter.
5. *Anticipatory care.* Take the opportunity to discuss the benefits of weight reduction and smoking cessation. Always clarify the patient's understanding of the benefits first and then educate appropriately, countering incorrect knowledge and building on the positive aspects of improving her lifestyle. Check to see if she wishes to act on either of these issues. If she is in agreement, formulate a plan with the patient and end the consultation with a specific target. Offer leaflets to support your advice. Arrange appropriate follow-up support, which may involve referrals to practice nurses, dieticians or specific self-help groups. If she declines your advice, clarify her reasons. Counter any ill-founded reasons. Explain that stopping smoking and weight reduction are the two most important actions she can take to achieve a healthier lifestyle, with stopping smoking being by far the more important. Focus on any relevant family history to help support your argument. Remember, it is your task to educate and inform your patient, but it is her right to decide whether to accept your advice or not.

6. Finally, it would be appropriate to take her blood pressure in view of her increased cardiovascular risk related to smoking and obesity and to exclude glycosuria in view of her obesity.

Scenario 11 (John Sutton)

Question 34

(Identify the most useful preventive opportunities that are present at this consultation and explain how you would proceed to act on them.)

Mr Sutton has an increased risk of ischaemic heart disease (IHD) as he is a smoker and his father had a MI at a relatively young age.

First, you need to explore Mr Sutton's views on this risk. Tell Mr Sutton you have noticed from the notes that his father has had a heart attack. Ask him if he is aware that this places him at a potentially higher risk of heart disease and, if this has been discussed with him previously. If it has, you will need to modify your response accordingly. If not proceed as follows.

- Clarify/probe his understanding of the genetic risk and educate if appropriate.
- Reassure him that it is possible to reduce this risk. Being positive will help enlist his support to alter lifestyle risk factors.
- You need to inform him of the single most important action he must take now, i.e. stop smoking.
- Check that he understands the harmful effects of smoking, and educate on the benefits of stopping as necessary. Concentrate on the benefits that are most relevant to Mr Sutton, i.e. the reduced risk of IHD.
- Counter any ill-founded justifications to continue smoking.
- Confirm his decision. Remember, it is his right to decide whether to accept your advice or not.

If he agrees to attempt to stop smoking, proceed as follows:

- Agree a plan. This should consist of a realistic target with appropriate follow-up to offer continuing support.
- Consider enlisting the help of his wife, especially if she smokes.
- Is there a 'stop-smoking' clinic he might wish to attend?
- Does he wish to use nicotine patches or chewing gum to reduce his craving?
- Later, if no progress is being made, alternative interventions such as acupuncture and hypnotherapy could be considered.

There are two other opportunities that you could consider today, if time is available and Mr Sutton is still receptive. However, you should avoid information overload and should not detract from the main message.

- Advise him to take regular exercise that makes him break out in a sweat 2–3 times a week, for 30–45 minutes. Explain that this will improve and maintain a satisfactory circulation of blood to the heart.
- Although his BMI is not raised, advice on a healthy diet would still be appropriate. Consider giving him a leaflet. Offer to check his serum lipids. You may need to explain the link between raised serum lipids and IHD. The results of these can be given at his follow-up appointment.

Finally, offer a summary of your advice, highlighting the importance of stopping smoking.

11

Assessing and enhancing consultation performance

Robin C. Fraser

No practitioner, however senior, who has
watched a video of themselves consulting
could be fully satisfied (van Zwanenberg,
1998).

Throughout this book it has been emphasized that the core attribute of
any clinician is the ability to perform satisfactorily in consultation with
patients. Furthermore, the General Medical Council (GMC) has identified
the acquisition of basic clinical method as a central objective of undergraduate medical education (GMC, 1993). Although your clinical teachers,
both in hospital and general practice, will assist you to acquire the
appropriate range of clinical competences, the GMC has also advised
medical schools to encourage and equip students to undertake more
responsibility for their own learning and professional development. Thus:

> A key aspect of the supervisor's task should be to help students to
> develop skills in diagnosis in respect of their own performance, so that
> when they leave college they will be capable of self-monitoring and
> improvement (Stones, 1994).

Chapter 10 provided you with a set of challenges to determine the
extent to which you are familiar with what you are required to do in
consultations with patients. This chapter will outline a systematic
approach to the analysis of your own global consultation performance, to
help enlighten you as to how you actually perform in real consultations
with patients. The latter part of this chapter will provide you with a
selection of specific actions you can take to assist you in overcoming any
identified weaknesses across the whole range of the component consultation competences contained in Chapter 2.

The approach outlined in this chapter has been shown to be highly
regarded by medical students (McKinley et al., in press). It can most
conveniently be applied to video recordings of your own consultations
(with the prior approval of the patients concerned); alternatively, you
could team up with a fellow student (or registrar) and take turns in
assessing each other's 'live' and/or video-recorded consultations.

Essential components of educational assessment

First, it might be helpful to introduce you to the essential components of educational assessment of performance.

Frequently, the term 'assessment' is (mis)understood as always referring to an 'examination'. In the current context, the term refers to educational or formative evaluation as a means of initially determining current capability.

> Formative evaluation emphasizes growth and development. [It] also implies analysis and diagnosis and I prefer the term diagnostic evaluation. Diagnostic evaluation should provide continuous feedback to students in a more analytical way than is usually the case (Stones, 1994).

There are three essential components of educational assessment or diagnostic evaluation:

- A test of performance
- An educational diagnosis
- An educational prescription.

In clinical medicine the most appropriate test of performance is the clinical consultation, in which a doctor has to respond to the wide range of challenges presented by different patients. The extent to which individual doctors can respond appropriately will determine their respective levels of clinical competence.

The next step is to undertake a diagnostic evaluation in order to arrive at an educational diagnosis. At its most simple level, this means identifying particular consulting strengths and weaknesses. (The ultimate goal should be to collate particular component strengths and weaknesses in order to produce an integrated diagnosis that accurately reflects and prioritizes the doctor's capabilities.) To do this, it is necessary to assess the doctor's performance against a set of explicit and validated criteria.

The third step is to formulate an educational prescription, i.e. a set of specific, practical and prioritized suggestions as to how a doctor can overcome any identified weaknesses.

It is a relatively easy task to recognize what is done well or badly in consultations. It is not at all easy, however, to identify omissions – i.e. what a doctor has not done when it should have been done. Most difficult of all – even for experienced clinical teachers – is the ability to formulate educational diagnoses and educational prescriptions. Accordingly, I would suggest that you begin the process of self-assessment by identifying your particular weaknesses (whilst noting your strengths); you should then consult the list of suggested actions that can be taken to assist in overcoming them (see later in this chapter).

A systematic approach to assessing your own consultation performance: the practical steps

This is based on the application of some of the components of the Leicester Assessment Package (LAP) (Fraser, 1994; Mulholland *et al.*, 1992).

Step 1

Familiarize yourself with:

- The required consultation categories and component competences (see Chapter 2), as these are the explicit criteria against which you will judge your performance.
- The criteria for the allocation of grades (see Figure 11.1). These descriptors will help you to assess your level of achievement and progress.

There is no need to commit these criteria to memory. You are advised, however, to have copies of both sets of criteria available for reference as you undertake Step 2.

The following descriptions of performance can be used as yardsticks of levels of achievement.

Grade	Criteria
A	Consistently demonstrates mastery of all components: the criterion performance.
B	Consistently demonstrates mastery of most components and capability in all.
C+	Consistently demonstrates capability in almost all components to a high standard and a satisfactory standard in all.
C	Demonstrates capability in most components to a satisfactory standard: demonstrates minor omissions and/or defects in some components. Duration of most consultations appropriate.
D	Demonstrates inadequacies in several components but no major omissions or defects.
E	Demonstrates several major omissions and/or serious defects; clearly unacceptable standard overall.

Figure 11.1 Assessment of consultation performance: criteria for the allocation of grades

Step 2

- Observe yourself consulting on video.
- Record details of your performance on the LAP Assessor's Recording Form (see Figure 11.2). Use one form for each consultation or part consultation you assess. As you observe the consultation, make a conscious effort to determine which component consultation competences are challenged and, if so, how you actually responded compared with how you should have responded.

At several stages of the consultation, if appropriate, it will often be useful to stop the videotape and ask yourself a number of questions as follows:

- At the end of initial history taking:
  - What were my diagnostic hypotheses at this stage?
  - Why had I erected them?
  - What physical examination should I have carried out and why?
- After any physical examination:
  - How had my findings affected my thoughts?
- At the end of the consultation:
  - Why did I choose my management plan?
  - Did I overlook any opportunistic preventive initiatives?

Hopefully, the answers to these questions will provide you with insights into the thought processes you have used (or not used) to underpin your actions. In this way, you will gain further and valuable insights into your capabilities with regard to the selective gathering, interpretation and application of information in history taking, physical examination and management.

Step 3

- Allocate a grade in each box to reflect your judgement of your own level of performance in each consultation category challenged, and for your overall consultation performance. Remember the relative weightings of the consultation categories; the most important being interviewing/history taking, patient management and problem solving (see Chapter 2 and Fig 11.1).

Step 4

- Make a list of the specific LAP component competences you judge to be your weaknesses. (You may also wish to make lists of your consultation strengths.)
- Consult the list of specific strategies for improvement to help correct identified weaknesses (see following section).
- Take the necessary action(s).

© THE LEICESTER ASSESSMENT PACKAGE: ASSESSOR'S RECORDING FORM

CANDIDATE ______________ ASSESSOR ______________ DATE ________

* If particular parameter does not apply to a consultation write N/A (not applicable).

Brief clinical details	Start time	End time	Duration
			Mins

CONSULTATION CATEGORY	POSITIVE FEATURES	WEAKNESSES/OMISSIONS	GRADE OF PERFORMANCE
Interviewing/history taking			
Physical examination			
Patient management			
Problem solving			
Bahaviour/relationship with patients			
Anticipatory care			
Record keeping			
Notes on overall performance (e.g. particular strengths/ weaknesses)			
Specific strategies for improvement			OVERALL

Figure 11.2 The Leicester Assessment Package: assessor's recording form

By repeating this process with multiple consultations you will not only become more familiar with the process, but also more proficient at self-assessment and enhancement of your consulting performance – a habit which should be continued throughout your professional career.

Strategies to help overcome consultation weaknesses

In this section are listed all LAP component consultation competences (with the exception of record-keeping). Underneath all of them are one or more suggestions for actions that could be taken to help readers to enhance their capabilities in respect of each listed consultation competence. The suggestions represent the consensus view of clinical academic staff and some practice clinical teachers associated with the Department of General Practice and Primary Health Care, University of Leicester. Although not exhaustive, the strategies for improvement reflect the contents of all the chapters in this book.

Interviewing/history taking

Introduces self to patients
- Always ensure the patient knows who you are and why you are there.

Puts patients at ease
- Welcome the patient – mention the patient's name, establish eye contact, give indication where to sit.

Allows patients to elaborate presenting problem fully
- Start with open questions, e.g. 'What can I do for you?', 'How can I help?', 'Tell me in your own words about . . .'.
- Use prompts as appropriate.
- At this stage, resist the temptation to interrupt.

Listens attentively
- Demonstrate to the patient that you are listening, for example by eye contact, nodding, etc.
- Try to understand the message that the patient is trying to convey.
- Don't displace the listening task by formulating the next question.

Seeks clarification of words used by patients as appropriate
- If you don't understand what the patient means, don't be afraid to ask for explanation/clarification.
- Don't assume the patient's use and understanding of medical or technical terms always correlates with your understanding of such terms, e.g. 'cystitis', 'constipation', etc.

Phrases questions simply and clearly

- Don't use jargon.
- Avoid using leading and/or double questions.
- Tailor questions to the patient's level of understanding.
- Ensure the patient can hear you by, for example, speaking louder to patients with reduced hearing – most often the elderly.

Uses silence appropriately

- Try to tolerate the discomfort of appropriate silences; for example, if the patient is having difficulty in telling his story and/or is distressed, allow him time to compose himself.

Recognizes patient's verbal and non-verbal cues

- Be aware of, and sensitive to, apparently incongruous or mismatched language or behaviour by patients; e.g., patients may say one thing but their body language might indicate another, the infrequent attender with an apparently trivial presentation, etc.
- Always consider the patient's demeanour and mood – happy or sad, tense or relaxed, angry or embarrassed, etc.

Identifies patient's reasons for consultation

- In every consultation you must be satisfied that you have established the patient's reason for the consultation. The answers to the following three questions need to be elicited: Why have you come? What do you think is wrong with you? What do you want me to do about it? Sometimes, you may have to ask these questions explicitly.
- Elicit the patient's concerns and expectations in every consultation; this may require gentle but persistent probing/questioning.

Elicits relevant and specific information from patients and/or their records to help distinguish between working diagnoses

- Prior to the consultation, always scrutinize the patient's record to elicit previous patterns of illness behaviour, individual and family circumstances, significant previous medical history (including current medication) and date and reason for most recent consultation.
- Always clarify the presenting complaint(s) first, then seek relevant associated features.
- Consciously identify in your mind the key, i.e. diagnostic, symptoms of each of your working diagnoses.
- Use focused questions to fill gaps in the information you are attempting to gather.

Considers physical, social and psychological factors as appropriate

- Always bear in mind the triple diagnosis.

- When satisfied that physical disease is present, always consider its impact on the social and psychological well-being of the patient.
- Consider the impact of other social and psychological factors on the patient – family, job, etc.

Exhibits well-organized approach to information gathering
- Use the hypotheticodeductive model in a systematic way.

Physical examination

Performs examination and elicits physical signs correctly and sensitively
- Become familiar with the appropriate technique of any part of the physical examination that was judged to be faulty – by reading about it, asking a tutor to demonstrate it, etc. – and then practise it under supervision.
- Ask patient's permission to carry out the examination, especially 'intimate' examinations.
- Appropriately expose the part(s) to be examined with due sensitivity to the patient.
- Give an explanation of what you are doing to the patient.

Uses the instruments commonly used in general practice in a competent and sensitive manner
- Familiarize yourself with the instruments incorrectly used (specify which), and practise their use under supervision.

Patient management

Formulates management plans appropriate to findings and circumstances in collaboration with patients
- Remember to apply RAPRIOP:
  Reassurance and explanation:
  Provide every patient with a basic explanation of your thoughts then try to reach a shared understanding of the nature of the problem and what can be done about it
  Whenever possible, link with the patient's reasons for consultation.
  Advice:
  Focus on areas of the patient's responsibility and what the patient can and/or should do.
  Prescription:
  Be consciously aware of the reasons for anything you prescribe
  Always consider the major side-effects and/or interactions
  If in doubt, don't guess; consult the BNF
  Provide adequate explanation to patients how prescribed items should be taken and their expected impact; include principal side-effects to be expected.

Referral:
Remember to consider the need for referral and consciously be aware of the reasons for and against any potential referral, whether to hospital, other members of the Primary Health Care Team, etc.
Investigation:
Remember to consider the need for investigation and consciously be aware of the reasons for and against any potential investigation.
Observation and follow-up:
Gear follow-up to the natural history of the condition you are dealing with
Remember the application of 'open' follow-up.
Prevention:
Remember to provide preventive advice relating to the problem(s) presented.

Makes discriminating use of investigations, referral and drug therapy
Covered above.

Is prepared to use time appropriately
- When the clinical picture is uncertain, it is sometimes appropriate to choose to defer decision-making until the clinical picture clarifies. (Sometimes the correct thing to do is apparently to do nothing.)

Demonstrates understanding of the importance of reassurance and explanation and uses clear and understandable language
- Don't use jargon.
- Tailor explanation to the level of the patient's understanding.
- Provide information in 'small packages', particularly if it is distressing or complex.
- Sometimes it may be appropriate to ask patients to tell you their understanding of the management plan and what they are to do. You may have to ask the patient 'Have you understood what I said?' or 'Is there anything else you would like to ask about what I have said?'.

Checks patients level of understanding
Covered above.

Arranges appropriate follow-up
Covered above.

Attempts to modify help-seeking behaviour of patients as appropriate
- Be prepared to advise patients on appropriate use of clinical services.

Problem solving

Generates appropriate working diagnoses or identifies problem(s) depending on circumstances

- Where possible, try to erect specific pathological, physiological and/or psychosocial diagnoses. If not possible, try to identify specific problems. Consider whether the PDI and sieves could assist in generating appropriate hypotheses.
- Ensure diagnostic hypotheses match your PDI.
- In erecting any single hypothesis, consciously test it against information for and against, then try to identify and fill any gaps.
- Generate a justifiable list under headings of 'Most likely' and 'Less likely but important to consider': actively consider whether every diagnosis should be present.
- Be prepared to reject diagnoses for which there is little or no support.
- Do not 'close' too early, i.e. jump to premature diagnostic conclusions.

Seeks relevant and discriminating physical signs to help confirm or refute working diagnoses

- Always assess whether the patient looks well or ill, particularly in children, and consider how this might influence your working diagnoses.
- Consciously ask yourself what the diagnostic physical signs for each of your working diagnoses are, and first focus your physical examination on eliciting their presence or absence.

Correctly interprets and applies information obtained from patient records, history, physical examination and investigations

- Take sufficient time to consider what the information you have gathered means, and how you can apply it. Don't be afraid to indicate to the patient that this is what you are doing.
- Think about the use of (interim) summarizing.
- Be prepared to check with books, colleagues, etc., particularly for single items of information.

Is capable of applying knowledge of basic, behavioural and clinical sciences to the identification, management and solution of patients' problems

- Remember you have a very substantial knowledge reservoir covering many subject areas.
- Before giving up, try to extrapolate from your knowledge of the principles of basic, behavioural and clinical sciences.
- Consider whether 'sieves' might help you to access your knowledge store.

Is capable of recognizing limits of personal competence and acting appropriately

- Nobody knows everything. It is an excellent professional attribute to be able to recognize the limits of your competence and then take the appropriate steps.
- When you recognize you have reached the limits of your competence, don't guess; seek appropriate help from colleagues, books, etc.

Behaviour and relationship with patients

Maintains friendly but professional relationship with patients with due regard to the ethics of medical practice

- Adopt friendly, professional behaviour and demeanour relevant to the circumstances of the individual patient and consultation.

Conveys sensitivity to the needs of patients

- Try to consider what it would be like to be in the patient's shoes, and respond appropriately within professional boundaries. Appropriate responses can include verbal and non-verbal acknowledgement of the patient's state, e.g. 'I can see you are angry; I can understand that', 'I can see why you are distressed about it'.

Demonstrates an awareness that the patient's attitude to the doctor (and vice versa) affects management and achievement of levels of co-operation and compliance

- In appropriate circumstances, a doctor has to be able to tolerate uncertainty. This may mean that, on occasions, the doctor will need to convey with confidence to the patient, with due regards to ethics, that a particular outcome is highly unlikely, although aware that no absolute guarantee can be given.

Anticipatory care

Acts on appropriate opportunities for health promotion and disease prevention

- Consider specific preventive interventions that could be made in any patient of the particular age and sex of the consulting patient.
- Always scrutinize the patient record to seek potential opportunities for preventive interventions in an individual patient.
- During consultations be alert for preventive cues, either verbal or non-verbal, e.g. nicotine-stained fingers/smell of alcohol.
- Remember there may be circumstances in the consultation or about a particular patient that might make a preventive intervention harmful even though otherwise indicated.
- Having identified legitimate preventive opportunities, be selective; normally restrict yourself to only one preventive action per consultation.
- Always establish the patient's motivation, i.e. readiness to change.

Provides sufficient explanation to patients for preventive initiatives taken

- In initiating your choice of preventive action, always provide the patient with an opening explanatory statement.
- Elicit patient's response (including level of awareness) and react accordingly.
- Be prepared, then or later, to provide evidence-based information on the reasons for the intervention.
- There is no point in continuing to try to alter the view of an informed patient who rejects the intervention.

Sensitively attempts to enlist the co-operation of patients to promote change to healthier lifestyles

- Try to agree a specific behaviour modification plan with the patient, which may include planned follow-up.
- Identify agreed targets; this may involve a series of interim targets.
- Throughout any preventive initiatives undertaken, be positive about benefits and be prepared to be supportive and to provide reinforcement.
- Offer continuing support and review of progress through follow-up.

Record keeping

See Chapter 2. Ways of achieving all criteria are self-explanatory.

Key points

- The core attribute of any clinician is the ability to perform satisfactorily in consultation with patients.
- All clinicians must develop the motivation and capability to monitor and enhance their own consultation performance as part of continuing professional development.
- Performance must be measured against an explicit and validated set of criteria in order to identify particular weaknesses (and strengths).
- Consultation performance can be enhanced by taking appropriate action to correct identified weaknesses.
- A systematic, valid and acceptable approach to the assessment and enhancement of consultation performance is set out in this chapter.

References

Fraser, R. C. (1994). *The Leicester Assessment Package*, 2nd edn. Glaxo Medical Fellowship.

General Medical Council (1993). *Tomorrow's Doctors. Recommendations on Undergraduate Medical Education*. London: General Medical Council.

190   Clinical Method

McKinley, R. K., Fraser, R. C., van der Vleuten, C. and Hastings, A. M. (in press). Formative assessment of the consultation performance of medical students in the setting of general practice using a modified version of the Leicester Assessment Package.

Mulholland, H., Fraser, R. C. and McKinley, R. K. (1992). The reliability of a limen referenced approach to the assessment of consultation competence in general practice: the Leicester Assessment Package. In *Approaches to the Assessment of Clinical Competence*, Part 1, pp. 192–8. Dundee: Centre for Medical Education.

Stones, E. (1994). Assessment of a complex skill: improving teacher education. *Assessment in Education*, 1(2), 235–51.

van Zwanenberg, T. (1998). In *GP Tomorrow* (J. Harris and T. van Zwanenberg, eds.). Abingdon: Radcliffe Medical Press.

Appendix: The detailed contribution of general practice to undergraduate medical education and to the attributes of the independent practitioner

The General Medical Council (GMC) is the body responsible for laying down the overall standard which students must achieve to pass the Qualifying (Final) Examinations in British medical schools. From time to time the GMC issues a detailed set of recommendations, on the basis of which undergraduate curricula and qualifying examinations are constructed. The latest *Recommendations* (GMC, 1993) list 27 educational objectives (of which 12 describe required knowledge, 3 describe required skills and 12 describe required attitudes).

The following are the 24 objectives selected from the GMC's original list which I believe general practice – and this book – can most particularly help a student to achieve (the letters used to denote each objective are those used in the original GMC list):

1. To acquire knowledge and understanding of:
   a. the *range of problems* that are presented to doctors and the *range of solutions* that have been developed for their recognition, investigation, prevention and treatment;
   b. how *disease presents* in patients of all ages, how patients react to illness or to the belief that they are ill, and how illness behaviour varies between social and cultural groups;
   c. the *environmental and social determinants* of disease, the principles of disease surveillance and the means by which diseases may spread, and the analysis of the burden of disease within the community;
   d. the principles of *disease prevention and health promotion*;
   e. the principles of *therapy*, including
      i. the management of acute illness;
      ii. the actions of drugs, their prescription and their administration;
      iii. the care of the chronically ill and the disabled;

     iv. rehabilitation and community care;
     v. the amelioration of suffering and the relief of pain;
     vi. the care of the dying;
  f. *reproduction,* including
     i. pregnancy and childbirth;
     ii. fertility and contraception;
     iii. psychological aspects;
  g. *human relationships,* individual and community;
  h. the importance of *communication*, both with patients and their relatives and with other professionals, both medical and non-medical, involved in their care;
  i. ethical and legal issues relevant to the practice of medicine;
  j. the *organization, management and provision of health care* in the community, the economic and practical constraints within which it is delivered, and the audit process to monitor its delivery.

2. To acquire and demonstrate skills in:
  a. *basic clinical method,* including the ability to
     i. obtain and record a comprehensive history;
     ii. perform a complete physical examination, and assess the mental state;
     iii. interpret the findings obtained from the history and the physical examination;
     iv. reach a provisional assessment of patients' problems and formulate with them plans for investigation and management.

3. To acquire and demonstrate attitudes essential to the practice of medicine, including:
  a. respect for patients and colleagues that encompasses, without prejudice, diversity of background and opportunity, language, culture and way of life;
  b. the recognition of patients' rights in all respects, and particularly in regard to confidentiality and informed consent;
  c. approaches to learning that are based on curiosity and the exploration of knowledge rather than on its passive acquisition, and that will be retained throughout professional life;
  d. ability to cope with uncertainty;
  e. awareness of the moral and ethical responsibilities involved in individual patient care and in the provision of care to populations of patients; such awareness must be developed early in the course;
  f. awareness of the need to ensure that the highest possible quality of patient care must always be provided;
  g. development of capacity for self-audit and for participation in the peer-review process;
  h. awareness of personal limitations, a willingness to seek help when necessary, and ability to work effectively as a member of a team;

i. willingness to use his or her professional capabilities to contribute to community as well as to individual patient welfare by the practice of preventive medicine and the encouragement of health promotion;

j. ability to adapt to change;

k. awareness of the need for continuing professional development allied to the process of continuing medical education, in order to ensure that high levels of clinical competence and knowledge are maintained;

l. acceptance of the responsibility to contribute as far as possible to the advancement of medical knowledge in order to benefit medical practice and further improve the quality of patient care.

In its 1993 Report, the GMC also identified the following attributes that it believes *any* independent practitioner should possess. Those marked with an asterisk are the ones to which I believe that general practice – and this book – can make a particular contribution (** major contribution, * contribution).

1. *The ability to solve clinical and other problems in medical practice*, which involves or requires:
   a. an intellectual and temperamental ability to change, to face the unfamiliar and to adapt to change;**
   b. a capacity for individual, self-directed learning;**
   c. reasoning and judgement in the application of knowledge to the analysis and interpretation of data, in defining the nature of a problem, and in planning and implementing a strategy to resolve it.**

2. *Possession of adequate knowledge and understanding of the general structure and function of the human body and workings of the mind, in health and disease, of their interaction and of the interaction between man and his physical and social environment.* This requires:
   a. knowledge of the physical, behavioural, epidemiological and clinical sciences upon which medicine depends;*
   b. understanding of the aetiology and natural history of diseases;*
   c. understanding of the impact both of psychological factors upon illness and of illness upon the patient and the patient's family;**
   d. understanding of the effects of childhood growth and of later ageing upon the individual, the family and the community;**
   e. understanding of the social, cultural and environmental factors which contribute to health or illness, and the capacity of medicine to influence them.**

3. *Possession of consultation skills*, which include:
   a. skills in sensitive and effective communication with patients and their families, professional colleagues and local agencies, and the keeping of good medical records;**

b. the clinical skills necessary to examine the patient's physical and mental state and to investigate appropriately;**

c. the ability to exercise sound clinical judgement to analyse symptoms and physical signs in pathophysiological terms, to establish diagnoses, and to offer advice to the patient taking account of physical, psychological, social and cultural factors;**

d. understanding of the special needs of terminal care.*

4. *Acquisition of a high standard of knowledge and skills in the doctor's specialty,* which include:

a. understanding of acute illness and of disabling and chronic diseases within that specialty, including their physical, mental and social implications, rehabilitation, pain relief, and the need for support and encouragement;**

b. relevant manual, biochemical, pharmacological, psychological, social and other interventions in acute and chronic illness.*

5. *Willingness and ability to deal with common medical emergencies and with other illness in an emergency.**

6. *The ability to contribute appropriately to the prevention of illness and the promotion of health,* which involves:

a. understanding of the principles, methods and limitations of preventive medicine and health promotion;**

b. understanding of the doctor's role in educating families and communities, and in generally promoting good health;**

c. the ability to identify individuals at risk and to take appropriate action.**

7. *The ability to recognize and analyse ethical problems so as to enable patients, their families, society and the doctor to have proper regard to such problems in reaching decisions;* this comprehends:

a. knowledge of the ethical standards and legal responsibilities of the medical profession;*

b. understanding of the impact of medico-social legislation on medical practice;*

c. recognition of the influence upon his or her approach to ethical problems of the doctor's own personality and values.**

8. *The maintenance of attitudes and conduct appropriate to a high level of professional practice,* which includes:

a. recognition that a blend of scientific and humanitarian approaches is required, involving a critical approach to learning, open-mindedness, compassion, and concern for the dignity of the patient and, where relevant, of the patient's family;**

b. recognition that good medical practice depends on partnership between doctor and patient, based upon mutual understanding and trust; the doctor may give advice, but the patient must decide whether or not to accept it;**

c. commitment to providing high quality care; awareness of the limitations of the doctor's own knowledge and of existing medical knowledge; recognition of the duty to keep up to date in the doctor's own specialist field and to be aware of developments in others;**

d. willingness to accept review, including self-audit, of the doctor's performance.*

9. *Mastery of the skills required to work within a team and, where appropriate, assume the responsibilities of team leader,* which requires:

a. recognition of the need for the doctor to collaborate in prevention, diagnosis, treatment and management with other health care professionals and with patients themselves;**

b. understanding and appreciation of the roles, responsibilities and skills of nurses and other health care workers;*

c. the ability to lead, guide and co-ordinate the work of others.**

10. *Acquisition of experience in administration and planning,* including:

a. efficient management of the doctor's own time and professional activities;*

b. appropriate use of diagnostic and therapeutic resources, and appreciation of the economic and practical constraints affecting the provision of health care;**

c. willingness to participate, as required, in the work of bodies which advise, plan and assist the development and administration of medical services, such as NHS authorities and trusts, Royal Colleges and Faculties, and professional associations.*

11. *Recognition of the opportunities and acceptance of the duty to contribute, when possible, to the advancement of medical knowledge and skill,* which entails:

a. understanding of the contribution of research methods, and interpretation and application of others' research in the doctor's own specialty;*

b. willingness, when appropriate, to contribute to research in the doctor's specialist field, both personally and through encouraging participation by junior colleagues.*

12. *Recognition of the obligation to teach others, particularly doctors in training,* which requires:

a. acceptance of responsibility for training junior colleagues in the specialty, and for teaching other doctors, medical students, and other health care professionals, when required;**

b. recognition that teaching skills are not necessarily innate but can be learned, and willingness to acquire them;**

c. recognition that the example of the teacher is the most powerful influence upon the standards of conduct and practice of every trainee.*

Reference

General Medical Council (1993). *Tomorrow's Doctors*. General Medical Council.

(RCF)

Index

Make time for friends.
Make time for Debbie Macomber.

DEBBIE MACOMBER